TYPE 2 DIABETES
COOKBOOK

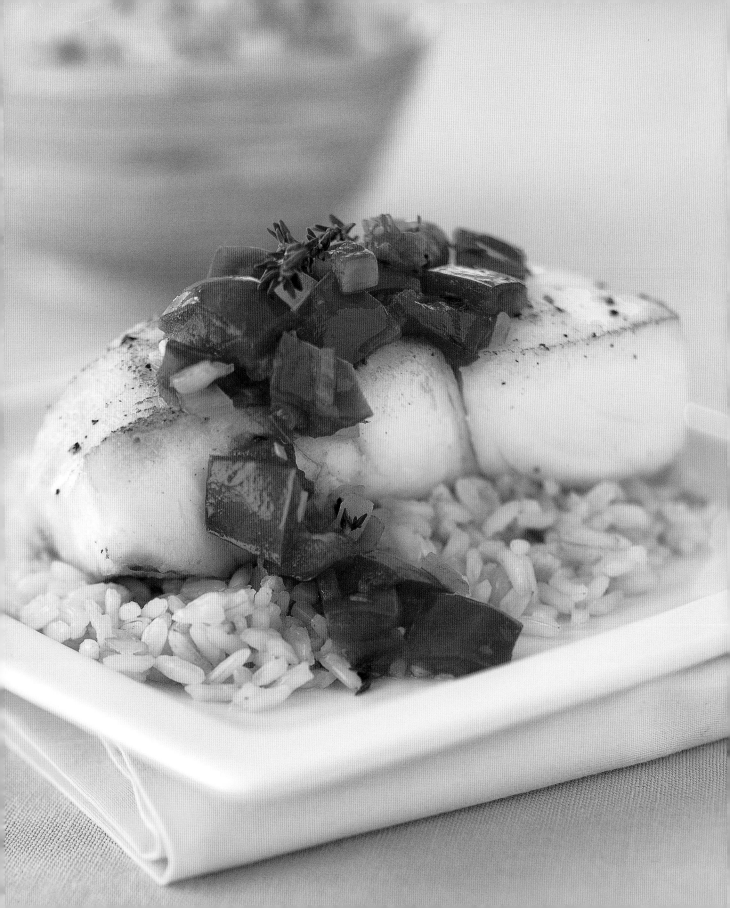

TYPE 2 DIABETES
COOKBOOK

RECIPES

Jackie Mills, R.D.

PHOTOGRAPHS

Sheri Giblin

WELDON OWEN

CONTENTS

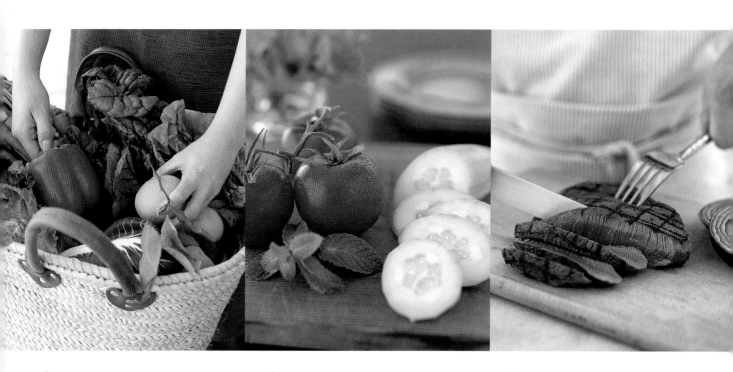

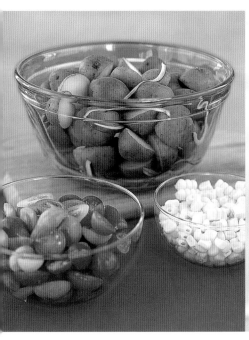
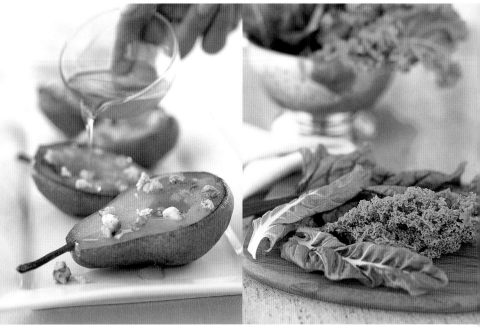

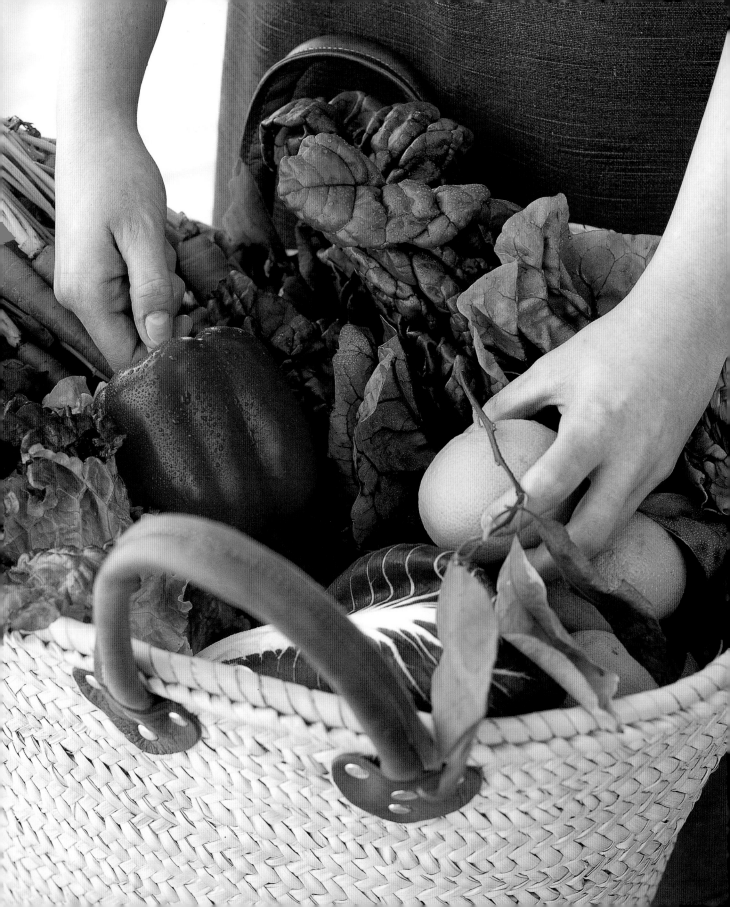

LIVING WELL WITH DIABETES

OUR HECTIC LIVES OFTEN PREVENT US FROM PREPARING HEALTHY MEALS AND TRULY ENJOYING THE PLEASURES OF EATING TOGETHER AS A FAMILY. Too often we turn to processed and fast foods because they are readily available and easy to put on the table. But that choice is making many of us, even our children, overweight.

Excess weight is the major cause of type 2 diabetes, a disease that is increasing dramatically among Americans, including more and more children. An estimated 18 million Americans now have type 2 diabetes and an additional 13 million have its precursor condition, prediabetes. Many don't know they have diabetes because the condition does not cause symptoms early on. The good news, however, is that type 2 diabetes can often be delayed, managed without medication, or even prevented—mainly by losing weight and exercising more.

This diverse collection of sixty recipes will help you and your family enjoy delicious, nutritious meals that are easy to prepare and can help you lose weight and better control your diabetes. Some of the recipes are so simple that your children can help you; they may even learn to make their favorite dishes themselves.

WHAT IS TYPE 2 DIABETES?

If your doctor has told you that you have type 2 diabetes or are at risk of developing it, he or she has recommended steps you can take to lower your blood sugar (glucose) level. For some people, losing weight, increasing activity, and eating a healthy diet are enough to help them avoid type 2 diabetes or the need for glucose-lowering medication.

Disease-fighting foods (facing page, clockwise from top left): green beans, blueberries, salmon steaks, and apples.

How type 2 diabetes develops

Type 2 diabetes develops from a mix of genes and lifestyle factors, mainly excess weight and lack of exercise, both of which cause the body to stop responding to insulin. Insulin is a hormone made by an organ called the pancreas to enable the body to use sugar for energy or store it as fat.

When the body fails to respond to insulin's effects, the pancreas makes more of the hormone, which then builds up in the blood. High levels of insulin in the blood, a condition called insulin resistance, can cause high blood pressure and harmful changes in blood fats like cholesterol. Insulin resistance—also known as metabolic syndrome—is the first step toward type 2 diabetes.

Prediabetes, the second step, occurs when the pancreas no longer makes enough insulin to move glucose into cells, and excess glucose builds up in the bloodstream. This gradual rise, if not diagnosed and treated, will eventually lead to type 2 diabetes.

The role of blood sugar

Because in its early stages type 2 diabetes causes no symptoms, it is often called a silent disease. For this reason, a third of people with type 2 diabetes don't know they have it.

But even without causing symptoms, high blood sugar can damage blood vessels and nerves. Over time, excess sugar can lead to blood circulation problems, heart disease, kidney failure, stroke from high blood pressure, and blindness. To avoid these complications, take any steps your doctor suggests to control your blood sugar. Your doctor will ask you to check your glucose level regularly.

Is your child at risk?

Until recently, few children or young adults developed type 2 diabetes. But the disease is becoming more common as American children eat too much and exercise too little. If your child is overweight, ask your doctor how to help him or her reach a healthy weight.

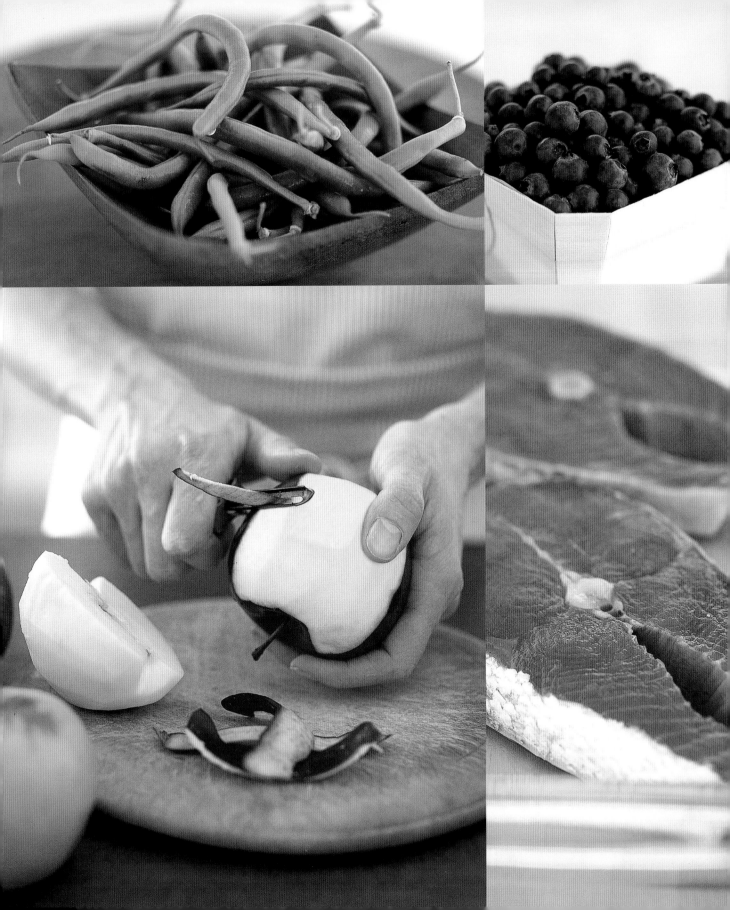

FIGHTING TYPE 2 DIABETES

Because type 2 diabetes tends to develop slowly over a period of several years, you can take steps to avoid it by adopting a healthy lifestyle. If you have been diagnosed with type 2 diabetes, these are the same measures your doctor will recommend to help you control your blood sugar and reduce your risk of complications from the disease.

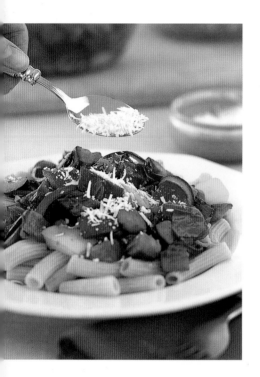

A healthy pasta dish such as Ratatouille Pasta (page 80) is a great choice for a main dish. A small amount of grated aged cheese adds flavor without too much fat.

Walking and playing outside (facing page) are smart ways for adults and kids to stay in shape. Take your kids—and yourself—to the park for fun and exercise.

Eat a healthy diet

A diabetes-fighting diet is heart-healthy, calorie-conscious, high in fiber and antioxidants, and low in harmful fats, added sugars, and salt. It is rich in whole grains, vegetables, legumes, and fruits, and replaces unhealthy fats from meats with healthy fats such as olive oil and omega-3 fatty acids from fish.

Lose those extra pounds

You can cut your risk of developing type 2 diabetes in half by losing as little as 7 to 10 percent of your current weight. If you do have type 2 diabetes, losing weight can make your body more sensitive to insulin, lower your blood sugar, and help you avoid the need for medication.

Don't smoke

Smoking impairs the body's usual sensitivity to the effects of insulin and raises the risk of high blood pressure, blood vessel damage, heart disease, and stroke.

Be active

Exercise is equally important. It lowers blood sugar by promoting weight loss and making the body more sensitive to the effects of insulin. Exercise also lowers blood pressure, improves blood cholesterol, reduces heart disease and stroke risk, and relieves stress—all of which help prevent complications from diabetes.

Try to engage in some kind of physical activity for 30 to 60 minutes every day. If you have been inactive for some time, talk to your doctor before starting an exercise program.

Control your blood sugar

If weight loss and exercise have not lowered your blood sugar to a healthy level, your doctor will prescribe sugar-lowering pills or insulin shots (page 11). You will be shown how to test your blood sugar regularly to see how well your diet, exercise, and medication are working. Careful monitoring of blood glucose is essential for avoiding complications.

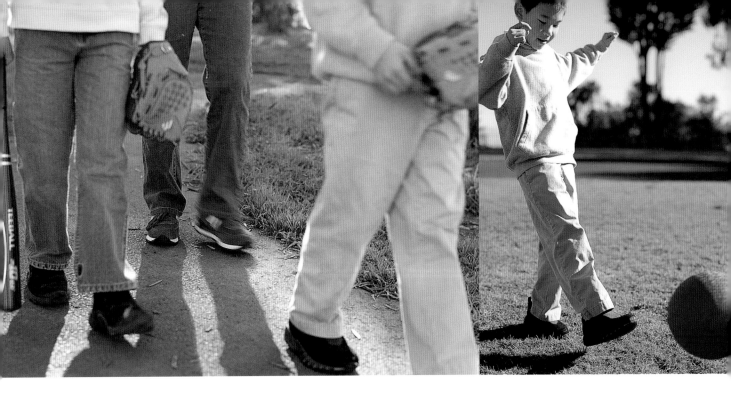

Lower your blood pressure

Many people with type 2 diabetes also have high blood pressure. Hypertension is especially harmful to people with diabetes because, like too much glucose in the blood, it can damage blood vessels and organs.

Have your blood pressure checked at each doctor visit. If your reading is higher than 120/80 mm Hg (high blood pressure is a reading above 140/90), the doctor will suggest steps you can take to lower it.

More and more American children and young adults are developing high blood pressure, mainly because they are overweight and inactive. If your child is overweight, have his or her blood pressure checked at each doctor visit, starting at age three.

Watch your cholesterol

If you're at risk of type 2 diabetes or already have it, you are likely to have an unfavorable blood cholesterol profile: total cholesterol above 200 mg/dL, HDL (good) cholesterol below 40, and LDL (bad) cholesterol above 100. While HDL helps keep your arteries open, LDL cholesterol can build up on artery walls. If you have an unhealthy cholesterol profile, your doctor will recommend lifestyle changes to improve it or prescribe a medication such as a statin.

Reduce stress

Stress heightens your diabetes and heart disease risks by raising blood glucose and blood pressure. Ask your doctor about effective ways to manage your stress.

DIABETES MEDICATIONS

To help you lower your blood sugar, your doctor may prescribe glucose-lowering pills. These drugs lower glucose either by increasing the pancreas's output of insulin, by making the cells more sensitive to insulin, by decreasing the liver's production of glucose, or by slowing the digestion of carbohydrates.

If sugar-lowering pills aren't helpful, your doctor may prescribe daily injections of insulin. This treatment may be temporary until you bring your glucose under control, or you may need to use insulin for the rest of your life. Your doctor will tell you how often you need to test your blood sugar to evaluate the success of your treatment plan.

SETTING NUTRITION GOALS

When it comes to eating a diet that can help you avoid type 2 diabetes and its complications, you have a lot of choices of healthy, nutritious foods. However, some basic guidelines apply.

For most people who have type 2 diabetes and those who are at risk of developing it, the bottom line to healthy eating is to eat less. Eat mostly high-fiber, plant-based foods such as whole grains, vegetables, legumes, and fruits and limit animal-based foods such as meat and full-fat dairy products, as well as salt and added sugars. Drink alcohol only in moderation.

Food is made up of carbohydrates, fats, and protein. Carbohydrates and fats are your body's main sources of fuel. Carbs should make up 45 to 65 percent of your daily calories, fats (mostly healthy, plant-based fats) 20 to 35 percent, and protein 12 to 20 percent.

HOW TO DISTRIBUTE YOUR DAILY CALORIES

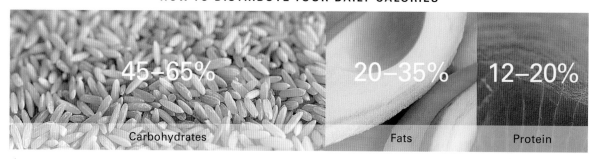

45–65%
Carbohydrates

20–35%
Fats

12–20%
Protein

CARBOHYDRATES

Carbohydrates are the sugars, starches, and fiber that make up plant foods such as fruits, vegetables, and whole grains. For people who are at risk of type 2 diabetes and those who have it, whole grains and fiber are especially beneficial because they do not increase blood sugar and insulin as much as do refined carbs like white bread and white rice.

45–65% OF DAILY CALORIES FROM CARBS

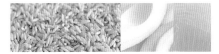

Healthy carbs

Whole grains—the seeds of grasses such as wheat, oats, rice, corn, rye, barley, millet, kasha, and quinoa— are linked to a lower risk of type 2 diabetes, heart disease, and stroke. They are rich in B vitamins, calcium, magnesium, and phosphorus.

Less-healthy carbs

When stripped of their outer husk, grains lose most of their nutrients and fiber. These processed, refined foods—such as white bread, white rice, and white pasta—are digested faster than whole grains and can quickly raise blood glucose.

Fiber

Fiber is the indigestible part of plant foods. Soluble fiber—found mainly in whole grains such as oats, rye, and wheat—is especially beneficial for people who have type 2 diabetes or who want to avoid it. It reduces blood sugar and the need for insulin and improves blood cholesterol.

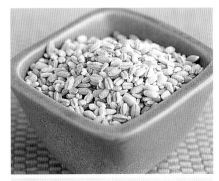

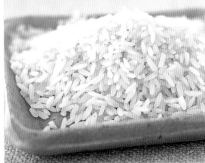

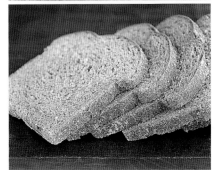

USING SUGAR SUBSTITUTES

Artificial sweeteners are carb-free, mostly calorie-free sugar alternatives. Used instead of sugar in dishes, they can help you lose weight or maintain a healthy weight. Sugar-rich foods tend to be high in calories and low in nutrients—and, most importantly, they raise blood glucose. Non-sugar sweeteners have no effect on blood glucose.

The most popular sugar substitutes are sucralose, aspartame, and saccharin. Sucralose is the only one whose sweetness doesn't change when it's heated and can therefore be used in cooking. But when using sucralose, and especially when baking, you may need to make adjustments such as increasing the amount of flour.

Keep in mind that using a sugar substitute in a recipe doesn't give you the freedom to overindulge. There are often lots of calories in the other ingredients, so it's still important to limit portion sizes.

HEALTHY FATS

20–35% OF DAILY CALORIES FROM FATS

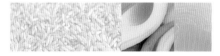

Fats in food provide energy, help the body absorb certain vitamins, make foods taste smooth, and make you feel full. Fats from seafood and oils from vegetables, nuts, and seeds provide health benefits that can protect your blood vessels and reduce your risk of type 2 diabetes and heart disease. These "unsaturated" fats are usually liquid at room temperature.

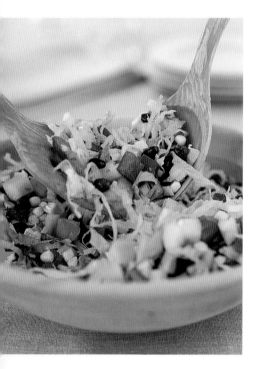

Avocado, Corn & Black Bean Salad
(page 51) offers a heart-healthy monounsaturated fat in the avocado, along with legumes and fresh vegetables.

Monounsaturated fats

These superhealthy fats come mainly from olive, canola, and peanut oils, most nuts, and avocados. They lower harmful LDL cholesterol in the blood, raise helpful HDL cholesterol, and cut triglycerides, easing the risk of type 2 diabetes and heart disease.

Polyunsaturated fats

Rich in omega-3 and omega-6 fatty acids, these fats lower cholesterol, although they may also lower helpful HDL cholesterol. Good sources are corn, sunflower, safflower, flaxseed, and soybean oils and fatty fish such as salmon and albacore tuna.

Plant sterols

Found in nuts, soybeans, seeds, and many other plant foods, these substances slow the absorption of dietary cholesterol and can lower total cholesterol and harmful LDL cholesterol in the blood. Look for salad dressings and tub margarines with added plant sterols.

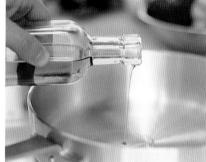

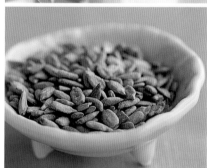

UNHEALTHY FATS

Some types of fats can harm your health, increasing your risk of type 2 diabetes, heart disease, blood vessel problems, and stroke. The most damaging fats are saturated fats and trans fats, which are usually solid or semisolid at room temperature. It's impossible to avoid all harmful fats because they occur in many foods, but it is wise to cut back.

Saturated fats

Found in meat, dark-meat poultry and poultry skin, butter, full-fat dairy products, coconut oil, and palm oil, these fats raise total cholesterol and LDL cholesterol, boosting the risk of heart disease and other diabetes complications. Make them less than 10 percent of your daily calories.

Trans fats

Vegetable oils can be hydrogenated, a process that extends the shelf life and maintains the flavor of foods. But these "trans fats," found in margarines, shortening, and many processed and fast foods, raise harmful LDL and total cholesterol.

Dietary cholesterol

Found in foods of animal origin—including egg yolks, liver, shellfish, full-fat dairy products, and meat and poultry—dietary cholesterol can raise blood cholesterol, but not equally in everyone and not as significantly as do saturated fats and trans fats.

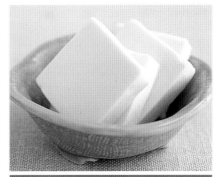

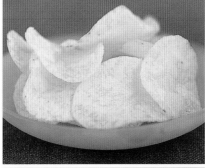

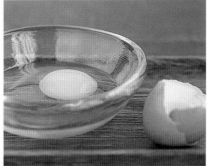

LIMITING FAT

When figuring your daily intake of fat (which should be no more than 30 percent of your total daily calories), consider the amount of fat eaten during the whole day, not just in one meal. If you have a rich breakfast, limit the amount of fat in your lunch or dinner that day. Some other tips:

• Make some meals meatless.

• Choose foods made with healthy plant-based fats, such as olive and canola oils, avocados, and nuts.

• Avoid fatty meats, full-fat dairy products, rich baked goods, and anything with hydrogenated oils or trans fats (check labels).

• Limit your cholesterol intake to less than 300 mg a day, or 200 mg if you have heart disease.

PROTEIN

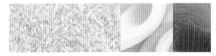

Protein, an essential nutrient found in both animal and plant foods, repairs tissues, builds muscle, and carries hormones and vitamins throughout the body via the bloodstream. Infants and children, because they are growing, have the highest daily protein needs pound for pound. Most adults consume far more protein than they need (see box at left).

HOW MUCH PROTEIN DO YOU NEED?

Adults need a surprisingly small amount of protein every day—only about 0.365 grams per pound of body weight. This means that if you weigh 140 pounds, your daily requirement for protein is 51 grams (140 x 0.365 = 51).

If you have advanced kidney disease, your doctor will ask you to limit your daily intake to 0.27 grams per pound of body weight.

Up to age 18, growing children require more protein, pound for pound, than adults. After age 18, their requirement is the same as that for adults. The chart below shows the average number of protein grams a child needs each day. Your child may need more or less than this amount depending on his or her weight.

1–3 years	— 16 grams
4–8 years	— 28 grams
9–13 years	— 46 grams
girls 14–18 years	— 55 grams
boys 14–18 years	— 66 grams

Animal proteins

Poultry, meat, milk, and eggs are rich in protein but can contain harmful fats and cholesterol (page 15). Look for lean meats and low-fat dairy products, remove the skin from poultry, and in recipes, replace one egg with two egg whites. Fish is an excellent heart-healthy protein.

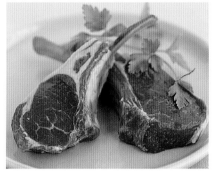

Plant proteins

Grains, beans and lentils, nuts, and some fruits and vegetables contain no cholesterol or unhealthy fats and are loaded with antioxidants and fiber. Vegetarians can get plenty of protein by combining whole grains, legumes, eggs, and dairy products.

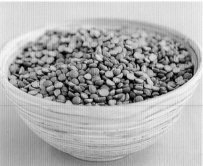

High-protein diets

Low-carbohydrate, high-protein, high-fat diets can result in rapid weight loss but in some people with diabetes may cause kidney problems; the long-term effects of these diets are unknown. Talk to your doctor before trying a high-protein diet.

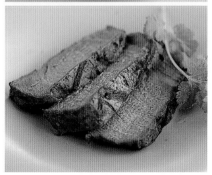

SODIUM

Sodium is linked to high blood pressure, common in people with type 2 diabetes. Although all people aren't equally sensitive to sodium's effects, doctors recommend getting less than 2,300 milligrams of sodium a day.

Where the salt hides

Most of us eat several times as much sodium as we need. Much of the salt comes from processed, packaged, and fast foods—not from the shaker. An easy way to limit salt is to eat more fresh foods such as fruits, vegetables, and whole grains. Select foods with less than 140 milligrams of sodium per serving, or 5 percent of the daily recommendation.

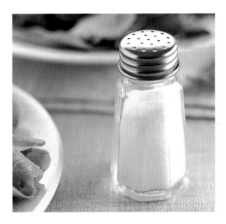

REPLACE SALT WITH NEW FLAVORS

Reprogram your taste buds to savor flavors other than salt. Experiment with alternative sodium-free flavorings such as herbs and spices; fresh lemon, lime, and orange juices; and garlic and onion powders. Salt-free seasoning blends are available to add to soups, stews, and casseroles.

EMPTY CALORIES

Most processed and fast foods are high in calories, which contribute to weight gain, and are digested more quickly than foods that are high in fiber. The result is an increased risk or worsening of type 2 diabetes.

Break the junk-food habit

Processed and fast foods are high in sodium and tend to be high in artery-clogging saturated and trans fats, low-quality carbs, and calories. Most American children drink more sugary soft drinks than water or milk, a trend linked to the rise in obesity and type 2 diabetes among children.

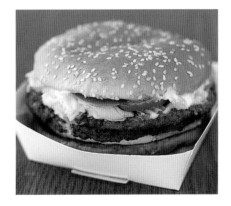

ALCOHOL'S EFFECTS

Although moderate drinking can reduce the risk of type 2 diabetes, heart attack, and stroke, doctors don't recommend that you start drinking for your health. If you drink alcohol, ask your doctor if it could interfere with any medications you are taking and how it could affect your blood sugar.

COUNTING YOUR CALORIES

To help you lose weight and better control your diabetes, your doctor may suggest different methods to limit calories, such as keeping track of the carbohydrates you eat in a day, with a specific number of grams in mind. Or you might use the traditional diabetic exchange system to plan your meals. Follow the steps in the next few pages to estimate your calorie allowance.

HOW TO FIND THE NUTRIENT VALUES IN EACH RECIPE

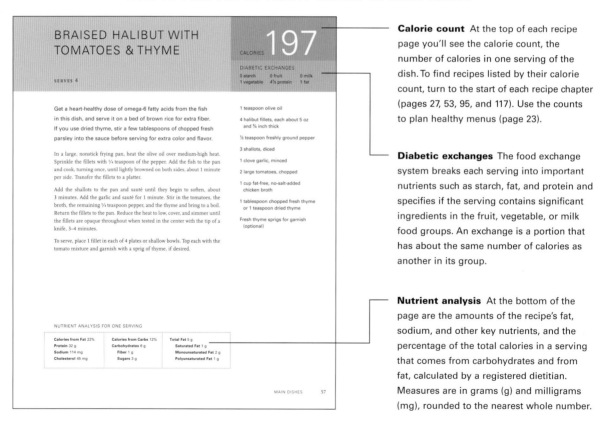

Calorie count At the top of each recipe page you'll see the calorie count, the number of calories in one serving of the dish. To find recipes listed by their calorie count, turn to the start of each recipe chapter (pages 27, 53, 95, and 117). Use the counts to plan healthy menus (page 23).

Diabetic exchanges The food exchange system breaks each serving into important nutrients such as starch, fat, and protein and specifies if the serving contains significant ingredients in the fruit, vegetable, or milk food groups. An exchange is a portion that has about the same number of calories as another in its group.

Nutrient analysis At the bottom of the page are the amounts of the recipe's fat, sodium, and other key nutrients, and the percentage of the total calories in a serving that comes from carbohydrates and from fat, calculated by a registered dietitian. Measures are in grams (g) and milligrams (mg), rounded to the nearest whole number.

HOW ACTIVE ARE YOU?

Your activity level and weight determine the amount of food you can eat. To lose weight, you need to burn more calories than you take in. The surest way to lose weight is to both increase your level of activity and reduce the amount of food you eat. Read the descriptions below to find the overall activity level that best describes yours.

Take your activity level and go to step 2 →

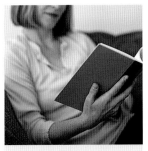

INACTIVE
Mainly sedentary most days of the week. Daily activities limited to driving, reading, watching TV, using the computer, and cooking with only rare, light exertion such as shopping.

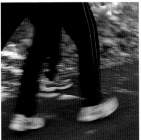

SOMEWHAT ACTIVE
Moderate activity throughout the week. Activities include light housework, leisurely walks, playing with children, climbing stairs at home, low-intensity sports such as golf or bowling.

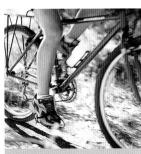

ACTIVE
Vigorous exercise several days a week. Activities include brisk walks, jogging, gardening, long bike rides, gym workouts, tennis or racquetball, swimming, dancing, or yoga.

ACTIVE KIDS ARE HEALTHY KIDS

Like adults, children who are overweight and inactive are at increased risk of type 2 diabetes. You can help your children avoid or delay type 2 diabetes—or manage it successfully if they have it—by encouraging them to be physically active at home, at school, and with their friends.

Make physical activity an important and fun part of every day—an hour at the very least is recommended for children. Limit their TV watching, video games, and other inactive forms of play. Sign your children up for sports they show an interest in and give them your support by attending games and other events.

Set a good example. When parents are active, children see exercise as a normal and important part of life. Plan active vacations and family events: take bike rides, hikes, and long walks. Go swimming, and spend time with your children playing catch and other games.

Why exercise is essential

Regular exercise can help you lose weight, maintain a healthy weight, control your blood sugar level, and manage your diabetes, possibly reducing your need for medication. Exercise may even help you avoid diabetes altogether. Other benefits of regular exercise include improved cholesterol levels, lower blood pressure, sounder sleep, more upbeat mood, increased alertness, and improved memory.

2 WHAT'S YOUR CALORIE COUNT?

To figure out how many calories you can eat each day to stay at your current weight, find your weight on the far left side of the chart below and locate your daily calorie allowance to the right in the column that corresponds to your activity level. To lose a pound a week, subtract 500 calories from your daily total.

To use the calorie count turn to page 23 →

LOSE WEIGHT SENSIBLY

The only sure way to lose weight is to burn more calories than you consume—that is, exercise more and eat less. A sensible approach is to lose about a pound or two a week—you're more likely to keep the weight off over the long term, giving you better control over your blood sugar and your diabetes.

Plan more meals and snacks around whole grains, vegetables, and fruits. And cut back on calories by watching portion sizes and lightening up on high-fat and sugary treats and fast foods. Here are some examples.

• To save 80 calories, have an apple instead of four shortbread cookies.

• To save 110 calories, eat half a cup (4 fl oz/125 ml) of low-fat frozen yogurt instead of a 1½-ounce (45-g) chocolate bar.

• To save more than 200 calories, order a 3-ounce (90-g) hamburger instead of a 6-ounce (185-g) one.

WEIGHT (in pounds)	INACTIVE	SOMEWHAT ACTIVE	ACTIVE
120	1500	1700	1800
130	1600	1800	1900
140	1700	1900	2100
150	1800	2000	2200
160	2000	2100	2400
170	2100	2300	2500
180	2200	2400	2700
190	2300	2500	2800
200	2500	2700	3000
210	2600	2800	3100
220	2700	3000	3300
230	2800	3100	3400
240	2900	3200	3600
250	3100	3300	3700
260	3200	3500	3900
270	3300	3600	4000
280	3400	3700	4100

CALORIES

YOUR CHILD'S CALORIE COUNT

To locate your child's approximate daily calorie allowance, find his or her age in the column on the left, then look to the right under "Girls" or "Boys." These allowances are general and are for moderately active children. Those who are very active or tall for their age need more calories. Children who are inactive or shorter than average need fewer.*

To use the calorie count turn to page 23 →

AGE	GIRLS	BOYS
3	1310	1400
4	1390	1480
5	1470	1560
6	1550	1640
7	1620	1730
8	1700	1810
9	1780	1920
10	1850	2010
11	1940	2130
12	2050	2270
13	2140	2450
14	2190	2640
15	2210	2820
16	2210	2940
17	2200	3010
18	2180	3040

CALORIES

HELP YOUR CHILD REACH A HEALTHY WEIGHT

You can help your child reach and maintain a healthy weight by providing nutritious meals and snacks and encouraging lots of physical activity. Some more tips:

• Give young children small portions to help them learn to eat only until satisfied. They can ask for seconds if they're still hungry.

• Offer more fiber-rich foods, such as fruits and vegetables and whole grains, and make them easily accessible for snacks.

• Switch from soft drinks and fruit drinks to water and low-fat milk.

• Don't keep high-fat, high-calorie foods such as chips and candy bars in the house.

• Serve at the table. Discourage eating while reading, studying, watching TV, or riding in the car.

• Eliminate bedtime snacks.

*For more specific guidelines, consult your child's doctor or a nutritionist.

COOKING FOR THE FAMILY

The best way to teach children the basics of good nutrition is to be a good role model and eat as many meals together as you can. Start when they're young, so they learn to make their own healthy food choices.

Make time for breakfast

Eating breakfast jump-starts your metabolism and helps you burn more calories throughout the day. It's especially important for children because it promotes proper growth and improves school performance. Easy, healthy breakfasts might be a bowl of an unsweetened high-fiber cereal with skim milk and a piece of fruit; a container of low-fat yogurt mixed with sliced fresh fruit and crunchy cereal; or hot oatmeal with dried fruit and a glass of skim milk.

Kid-friendly lunches

Encourage your kids to look beyond peanut butter and jelly sandwiches. If they get lunch at school, make sure the meals are low in fat, calories, and added sugars. If not, suggest the school offer healthier choices and eliminate high-calorie foods such as pizza, fries, chips, soft drinks, and candy bars. At home, try making sandwiches with whole-grain breads, lean meats and poultry, low-fat mayonnaise or mustard, and lettuce, tomato, and other vegetables.

SHOP SMART

Having healthy ingredients on hand—such as fresh vegetables and low-sodium canned broths, beans, and tomatoes—allows you to quickly assemble nutritious meals.

- Look for reduced-fat, fat-free, low-sodium, and sugar-free products, including low-fat cheeses and unsweetened high-fiber cereals.

- Stock plenty of fresh, frozen, and canned vegetables and fruits (without added sodium and sugar).

- Stay away from fatty and salty snack foods such as potato chips.

- Use olive and canola oils and soft or liquid margarines with plant sterols instead of stick margarines.

- Try to serve a few meatless meals every week.

Tips for cutting calories

Eat only when you're hungry.

Eat slowly (it takes 20 to 30 minutes to start feeling full).

Stop eating when you're full.

Begin meals with a large glass of water.

Choose a fruit or vegetable for a snack.

Reduce serving sizes of high-fat meats, desserts, and other high-fat foods.

Choose low-fat or no-fat cheeses, salad dressings, and bread spreads.

Use low-fat cooking methods such as baking, broiling, grilling, or steaming.

Use cooking sprays for frying and sautéeing.

Keep a food log to help you track how much you're eating.

PLANNING HEALTHY DINNERS

Preparing healthy dinners doesn't need to be time-consuming or difficult. As examples, we've combined dishes from this book into several simple menus for nutritious, satisfying dinners that you and your family will enjoy. What's more, in the following pages you'll find a number of special "kid-friendly recipes" designed to appeal to children.

AMERICAN (and kid-friendly)

Vegetable Noodle Soup	90 calories
Herb-Crusted Chicken	203 calories
Baby Carrots with Orange Glaze	65 calories
Banana-Berry Parfaits	101 calories
Total	459 calories

MEDITERRANEAN

Red Pepper & Provolone Crostini	83 calories
Snapper with Summer Squash & Tomato	203 calories
Creamy Polenta with Kale & Parmesan	131 calories
Baked Pears with Honey, Blue Cheese & Walnuts	112 calories
Total	529 calories

SOUTHWESTERN

Tomato & Red Bell Pepper Soup	66 calories
Avocado, Corn & Black Bean Salad	151 calories
Vegetable Enchiladas	242 calories
Grilled Pineapple with Orange-Cinnamon Glaze	69 calories
Total	528 calories

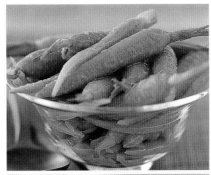

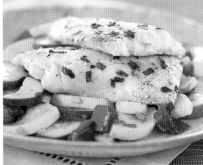

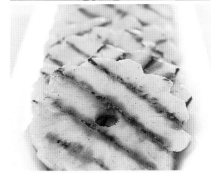

WATCH EVERYDAY PORTION SIZES

When you're trying to lose weight or stay at a healthy weight, limiting portion size is especially important. To help you eyeball portion sizes, try using the dimensions of your hand.

• Palm = 3 ounces (90 g) of meat, poultry, or fish

• Fist = 1 medium fruit or 1 cup (4 oz/125 g) of cut-up fruit

• Cupped hand = 1 to 2 ounces (30 to 60 g) of almonds or other nuts

• Thumb (base to tip) = 1 ounce (30 g) of meat or cheese

When checking the calories of a packaged food, be sure to note the serving size. There may be only 100 calories per serving, but if there are 4 servings in the package and you eat the whole package, you're consuming 400 calories. Likewise, with each recipe in this book, you'll find the calories per serving and the number of servings. If there are 4 servings and you eat half the dish, be sure to double the calorie count.

HEALTHY SNACKS TO KEEP ON HAND

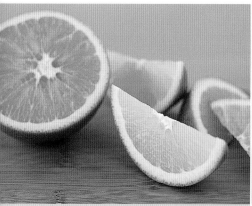

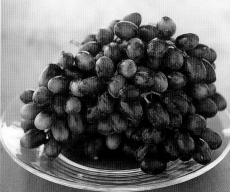

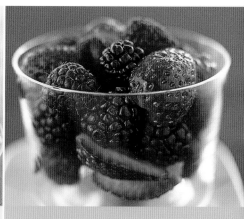

ORANGES
Peeled and pulled apart into segments or cut into wedges, oranges are vitamin C–packed breakfast favorites that help your body absorb iron.

GRAPES
A perfect low-calorie treat, grapes are 80 percent water with only 60 calories in a cup. Kids love them because they're sweet, juicy, and fun to eat.

BERRIES
These colorful, nutrient-dense fruits make great toppings for cereal and yogurt, add richness to smoothies, and freeze well and thaw quickly for a refreshing snack.

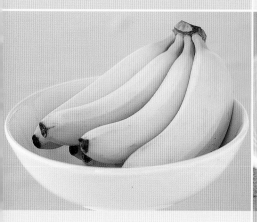

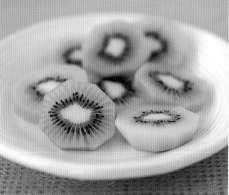

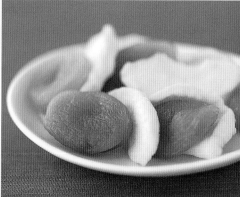

BANANAS
Bananas are neatly packaged by nature and fun to peel. Available year round, they are rich in healthy carbohydrates and easy to slip into a lunch box or sack.

KIWIFRUIT
Kiwifruit comes in its own serving cup: Just cut it in half and scoop out the flesh with a spoon. Or, for a nicer presentation, peel the skin and cut the flesh into slices.

DRIED FRUIT
When dried, fruits lose moisture and gain a longer shelf life. But dried fruits are much higher in calories and sugar than fresh ones, so watch portion sizes.

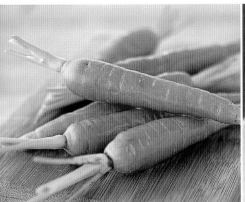

CARROTS

Rich in vitamin A and beta carotene, carrots are favorites of both children and adults. Eat them whole, cut into sticks, or shredded in salads.

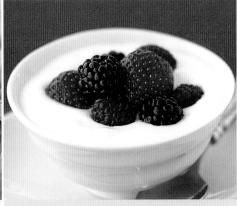

NONFAT YOGURT

Plain yogurt is an excellent source of bone-building calcium and one of the healthiest foods you can eat. Mix it with fruit for sundaes and shakes.

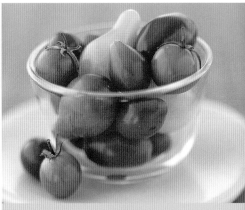

TOMATOES

Cherished in many cuisines, tomatoes are known cancer fighters. Keep the cherry and grape versions out in a bowl for snacking.

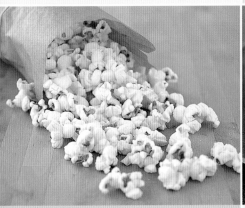

POPCORN

Air-popped popcorn is sugar free, fat free, low in calories, and high in fiber, making it an especially smart family treat. Add to dried fruit and nuts for a trail mix.

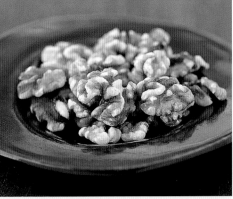

UNSALTED NUTS

Eating a handful of nuts a day is good for your heart. What's more, because nuts are so satisfying, they may even help you lose weight. Keep a variety on hand.

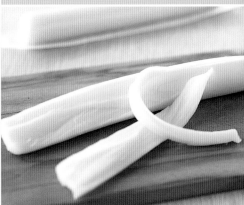

STRING CHEESE

Kids love string cheese—the pull-apart food—which makes it an easy way to supply them with calcium for their growing bones and teeth.

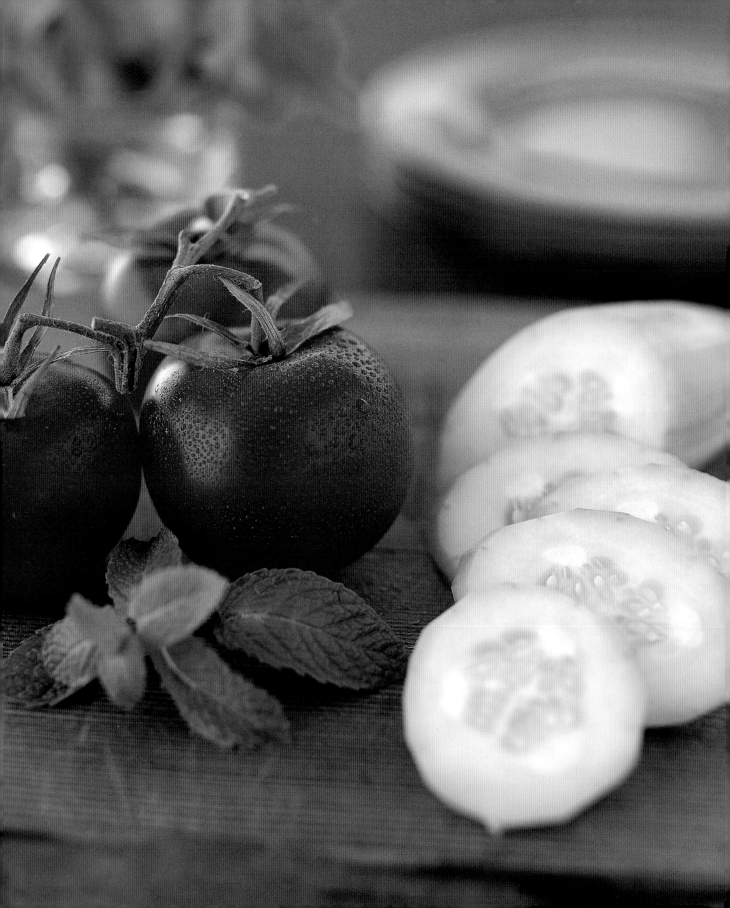

STARTERS, SOUPS & SALADS

CALORIES	
39c	SESAME SLAW, 48
54c	TOMATO & CUCUMBER SALAD WITH MINT PESTO, 44
66c	TOMATO & RED BELL PEPPER SOUP, 37
83c	ROASTED RED PEPPER & PROVOLONE CROSTINI, 31
90c	VEGETABLE NOODLE SOUP, 36
98c	SESAME NOODLE SOUP, 40
103c	BREAD SALAD WITH ROASTED RED PEPPERS, 47
105c	VEGETABLE PLATTER WITH LEMON-BASIL EDAMAME DIP, 35

CALORIES	
105c	SHRIMP & SWEET CORN SOUP, 39
106c	APPLE, RAISIN & ALMOND SALAD, 43
108c	CHICKEN SKEWERS WITH SESAME-SOY SAUCE, 28
118c	BULGUR SALAD WITH FENNEL & SPINACH, 50
132c	WHOLE-WHEAT PIZZA WITH MOZZARELLA & TOMATO, 32
151c	AVOCADO, CORN & BLACK BEAN SALAD, 51

Tomato & Cucumber Salad with Mint Pesto, 44

DIABETIC EXCHANGES

| 0 starch | 0 fruit | 0 milk |
| 0 vegetable | 2½ protein | ½ fat |

SERVES 6

1 lb (500 g) skinless, boneless chicken breast, cut into ¼-inch (6-mm) slices

Eighteen 6-inch (15-cm) metal or presoaked wooden skewers

2 teaspoons grated lime zest

¼ cup (2 fl oz/60 ml) plus 3 tablespoons fresh lime juice

¾ teaspoon dark sesame oil

2 cloves garlic, minced

2 tablespoons rice vinegar or white wine vinegar

1 tablespoon low-sodium soy sauce

1 teaspoon peeled and minced fresh ginger

⅛ teaspoon red pepper flakes

1 teaspoon olive oil

1 head Bibb lettuce, inner leaves left whole and larger leaves torn in half

Impress dinner guests with this delicate low-fat, Asian-inspired dish. The tangy fresh lime marinade is also excellent for grilled shrimp; marinate the shrimp for 15–20 minutes before cooking.

Thread the chicken slices onto the skewers. In a shallow dish, combine the lime zest, ¼ cup of the lime juice, ½ teaspoon of the sesame oil, and the garlic and stir to combine. Add the chicken skewers and turn to coat. Cover and refrigerate for 30 minutes.

Meanwhile, in a small bowl, combine the remaining 3 tablespoons lime juice and ¼ teaspoon sesame oil, the vinegar, soy sauce, ginger, and red pepper flakes. Stir the dipping sauce until well blended.

Preheat the broiler (grill) and position the rack 4–6 inches (10–15 cm) from the heat source. Lightly coat the broiler pan with the olive oil. Place the skewers on the rack and broil (grill), turning once, until the chicken is opaque throughout, 3–4 minutes per side. To serve, place the skewers on lettuce leaves and arrange on a serving platter with the dipping sauce. Serve hot.

NUTRIENT ANALYSIS FOR ONE SERVING

Calories from Fat 20%	**Calories from Carbs** 11%	**Total Fat** 2 g
Protein 18 g	**Carbohydrates** 3 g	**Saturated Fat** 0 g
Sodium 116 mg	**Fiber** 0 g	**Monounsaturated Fat** 1 g
Cholesterol 44 mg	**Sugars** 1 g	**Polyunsaturated Fat** 1 g

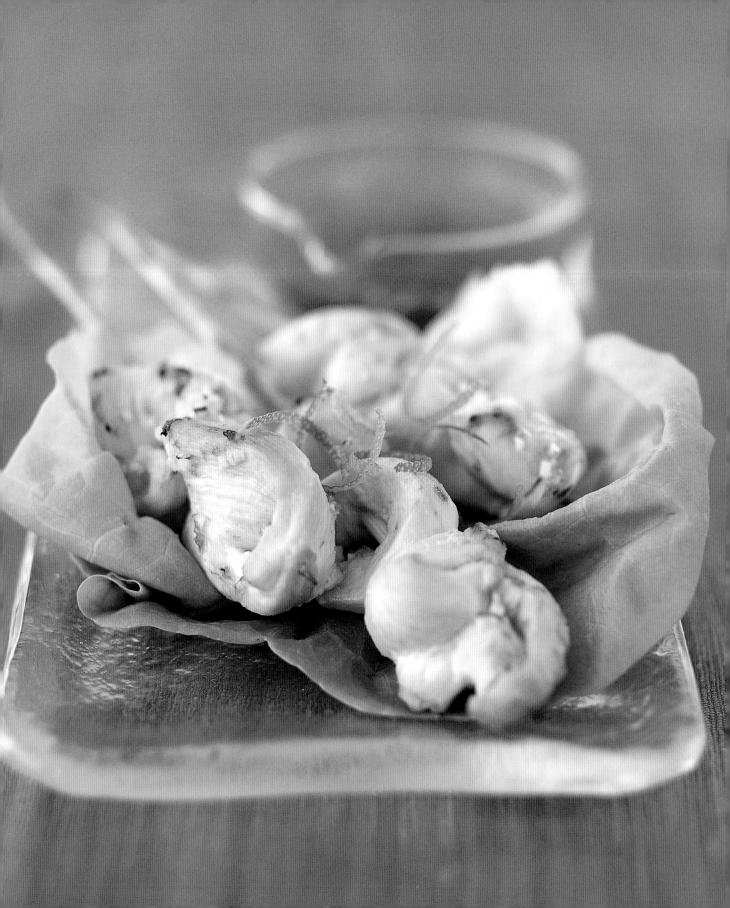

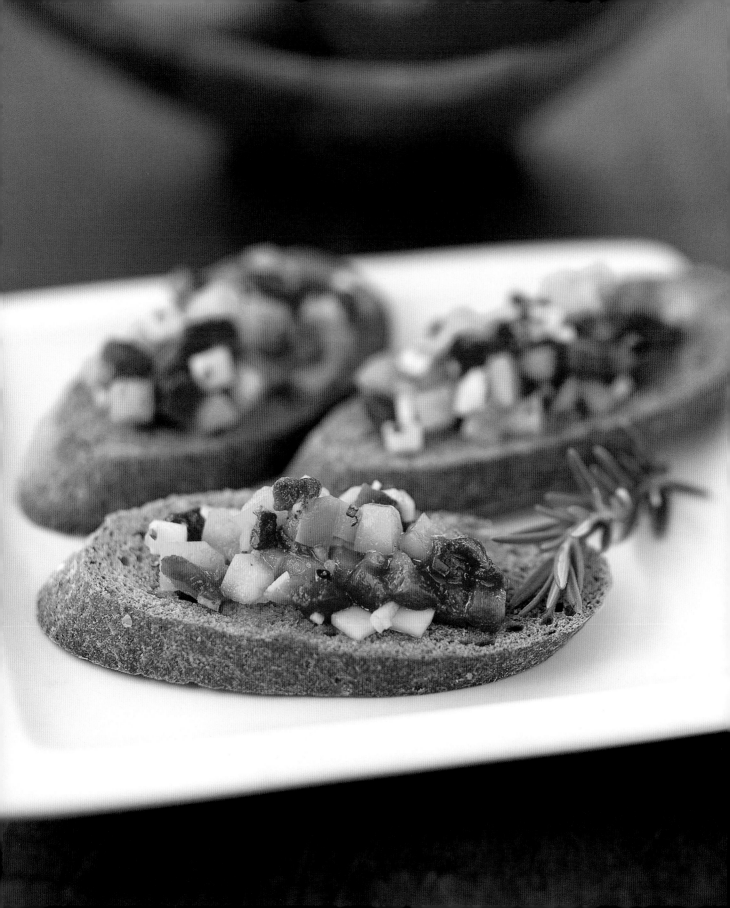

ROASTED RED PEPPER & PROVOLONE CROSTINI

CALORIES **83**

DIABETIC EXCHANGES

1 starch	0 fruit	0 milk
½ vegetable	0 protein	½ fat

SERVES 6

You can make the topping for the crostini ahead of time, but bring it to room temperature before serving for better flavor. Look for yellow tomatoes at your local market; they add color to the dish and contrast nicely with the red peppers.

Preheat the oven to 350°F (180°C). Arrange the bread slices in a single layer on a baking sheet and bake until lightly toasted, 8–10 minutes.

While the bread is toasting, in a bowl, combine the vinegar, olive oil, garlic, rosemary, and ground pepper and stir to mix well. Add the roasted red peppers, tomato, and cheese. Toss gently to coat. Spoon 1 tablespoon of the vegetable mixture onto each toasted baguette slice. Serve immediately.

18 slices whole-wheat (wholemeal) baguette, about ⅓ inch (9 mm) thick

1 teaspoon balsamic vinegar

1 teaspoon olive oil

1 small clove garlic, minced

1 teaspoon chopped fresh rosemary or 1 teaspoon crumbled dried rosemary

¼ teaspoon freshly ground pepper

½ cup (4 oz/125 g) roasted red peppers from a jar, drained and diced

1 small tomato, seeded and diced

1 oz (30 g) provolone cheese, diced

NUTRIENT ANALYSIS FOR ONE SERVING

Calories from Fat 24%	**Calories from Carbs** 62%	**Total Fat** 2 g
Protein 3 g	**Carbohydrates** 14 g	**Saturated Fat** 1 g
Sodium 137 mg	**Fiber** 4 g	**Monounsaturated Fat** 1 g
Cholesterol 3 mg	**Sugars** 2 g	**Polyunsaturated Fat** 0 g

WHOLE-WHEAT PIZZA WITH MOZZARELLA & TOMATO

SERVES 4   Kid-friendly recipe

- ¾ cup (4 oz/125 g) whole-wheat flour
- 1 teaspoon rapid-rise yeast
- ⅓ cup (3 fl oz/90 ml) plus 1 to 2 tablespoons warm water
- 1 teaspoon olive oil
- ¼ cup (1 oz/30 g) shredded part-skim mozzarella cheese
- 2 small plum (Roma) tomatoes, thinly sliced
- 1 tablespoon chopped fresh basil or 1½ teaspoons dried basil

Rapid-rise yeast makes this pizza dough ready in minutes. Just be sure to place the dough in a warm place to rise. Serve the pizza as an appetizer for four or as a light lunch for two. Try topping the crust with your favorite healthy ingredients.

In a bowl, combine the flour and yeast. Add ⅓ cup of the warm water and stir until blended. Add the remaining warm water, 1 tablespoon at a time as needed, until the dough forms a ball. Turn the dough out onto a lightly floured work surface and knead 4 or 5 times. Coat a large bowl with ½ teaspoon of the olive oil. Place the dough in the oiled bowl and turn to coat. Cover and let stand in a warm place until the dough has doubled in bulk, about 20 minutes.

Place a rack in the lowest position of the oven and preheat to 475°F (245°C). Using your fingertips, coat a 12-inch (30-cm) round pizza pan with the remaining ½ teaspoon olive oil. Press the dough into the pan, using your oiled fingertips to spread it to the edges. Bake for 5 minutes. Remove from the oven and, using tongs, turn it over on the pan, browned side up.

Sprinkle the crust evenly with the mozzarella. Top with the tomato slices and basil. Bake until the cheese is bubbly and the bottom is browned, 4–5 minutes. Cut into wedges and serve immediately.

NUTRIENT ANALYSIS FOR ONE SERVING

Calories from Fat 24%	**Calories from Carbs** 57%	**Total Fat** 3 g
Protein 6 g	**Carbohydrates** 19 g	**Saturated Fat** 1 g
Sodium 41 mg	**Fiber** 4 g	**Monounsaturated Fat** 1 g
Cholesterol 4 mg	**Sugars** 2 g	**Polyunsaturated Fat** 0 g

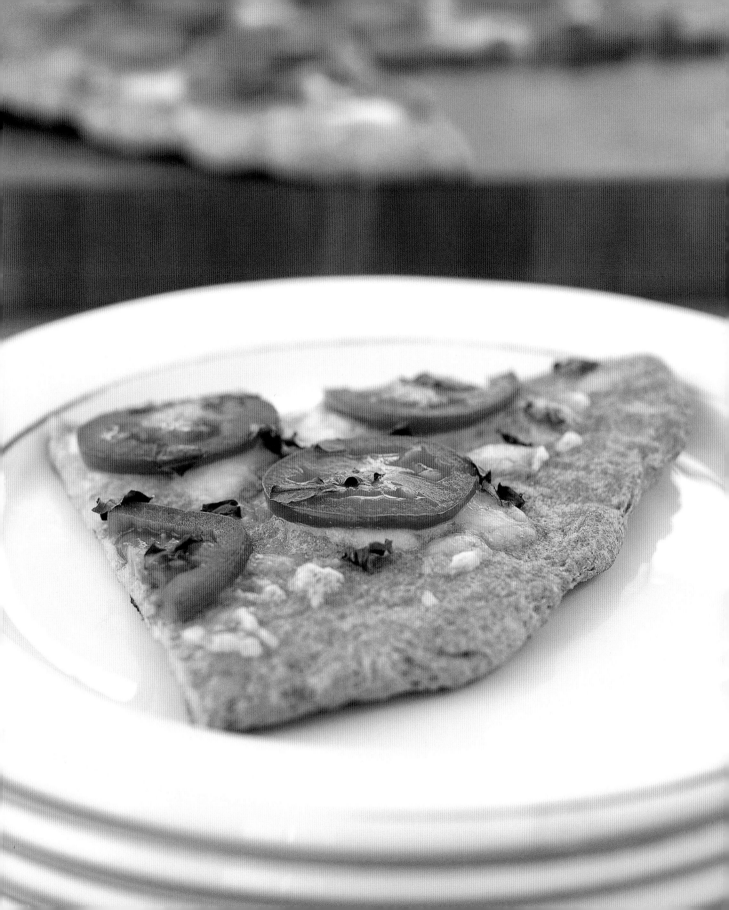

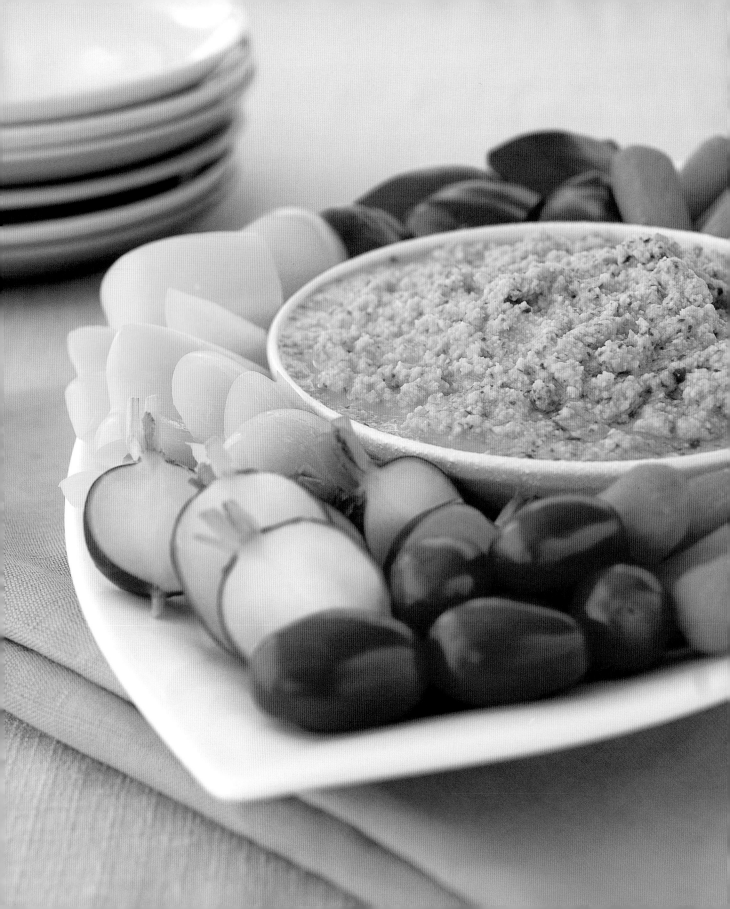

VEGETABLE PLATTER WITH LEMON-BASIL EDAMAME DIP

CALORIES 105

DIABETIC EXCHANGES

| ½ starch | 0 fruit | 0 milk |
| 1½ vegetable | ½ protein | ½ fat |

SERVES 6

Edamame—fresh soybeans that are picked before they fully mature—are an excellent source of fiber and protein. If they are unavailable, substitute an equal amount of thawed frozen baby lima beans or canned cannellini beans (rinsed and drained).

In a food processor or blender, combine the edamame, basil, lemon zest and juice, broth, and olive oil. Process until smooth. Transfer the dip to a serving bowl.

To serve, arrange the carrots, bell peppers, radishes, and tomatoes on a serving platter with the dip.

1½ cups (7½ oz/235 g) frozen shelled edamame (fresh soybeans), thawed

¼ cup (¼ oz 7 g) whole fresh basil leaves or 1 teaspoon dried basil

1 teaspoon grated lemon zest

2 tablespoons fresh lemon juice

¾ cup (6 fl oz/180 ml) fat-free, no-salt-added vegetable or chicken broth

2 teaspoons olive oil

2 cups (10 oz/315 g) baby carrots

1 red bell pepper (capsicum), cut into large bite-sized chunks

1 yellow bell pepper (capsicum), cut into large bite-sized chunks

1 cup (6 oz/185 g) small trimmed radishes

1 cup (6 oz/185 g) cherry tomatoes

NUTRIENT ANALYSIS FOR ONE SERVING

Calories from Fat 27%	Calories from Carbs 53%	Total Fat 3 g
Protein 5 g	Carbohydrates 14 g	Saturated Fat <1 g
Sodium 85 mg	Fiber 4 g	Monounsaturated Fat 1 g
Cholesterol 0 mg	Sugars 5 g	Polyunsaturated Fat <1 g

VEGETABLE NOODLE SOUP

SERVES 6   Kid-friendly recipe

- 2 oz (60 g) whole-wheat (wholemeal) or 50-percent whole-wheat wide egg noodles

- 2 teaspoons olive oil

- 1 yellow onion, chopped

- 1 carrot, peeled and chopped

- 1 celery stalk, chopped

- 5 cups (40 fl oz/1.25 l) fat-free, no-salt-added vegetable or chicken broth

- 1 zucchini (courgette), chopped

- 1 tomato, chopped

- 2 tablespoons chopped fresh parsley (optional)

- ¼ teaspoon freshly ground pepper

Make this soup in the summer, when there's a bumper crop of zucchini and tomatoes. Try stirring in other vegetables—a diced yellow squash or 2 cups (4 oz/125 g) fresh chopped spinach. For a complete meal, add cooked chicken or cannellini beans.

Bring a large pot three-fourths full of water to a boil. Add the noodles and cook until al dente, 10–12 minutes, or according to package directions. Drain the pasta thoroughly and set aside.

While the pasta is cooking, in a large saucepan, heat the olive oil over medium heat. Add the onion, carrot, and celery and sauté until the vegetables are softened, about 5 minutes. Add the broth and bring to a simmer. Cook, covered, until the vegetables are tender, about 10 minutes. Add the zucchini and tomato and return to a simmer. Cook, covered, until the zucchini is tender, about 3 minutes longer. Stir in the parsley (if using), the noodles, and the pepper and simmer for 1 minute longer. Ladle into individual bowls and serve.

NUTRIENT ANALYSIS FOR ONE SERVING

Calories from Fat 19%	**Calories from Carbs** 54%	**Total Fat** 2 g
Protein 6 g	**Carbohydrates** 13 g	**Saturated Fat** 0 g
Sodium 126 mg	**Fiber** 2 g	**Monounsaturated Fat** 1 g
Cholesterol 0 mg	**Sugars** 3 g	**Polyunsaturated Fat** 0 g

TOMATO & RED BELL PEPPER SOUP

CALORIES

66

DIABETIC EXCHANGES

| 0 starch | 0 fruit | 0 milk |
| 2 vegetable | 0 protein | ½ fat |

SERVES 6

Red bell pepper (capsicum) adds a touch of sweetness and extra antioxidants to this traditional tomato soup. Make it heartier by adding cooked whole-wheat (wholemeal) egg noodles or brown rice. If you have fresh basil, use it to give an even livelier flavor.

In a large saucepan, heat the olive oil over medium-high heat. Add the onion, bell pepper, and garlic and sauté until the vegetables are softened, about 5 minutes.

Add the tomatoes, their juices, and the broth and bring to a boil. Reduce the heat to medium-low and simmer, covered, for 25 minutes. Add the ground pepper and basil and cook for 5 minutes longer. Ladle the soup into individual bowls and serve immediately.

2 teaspoons olive oil

1 yellow onion, chopped

1 large red bell pepper (capsicum), chopped

2 cloves garlic, minced

Two 14-oz (440-g) cans no-salt-added whole tomatoes, drained and chopped, juices reserved

3 cups (24 fl oz/750 ml) fat-free, no-salt-added vegetable or chicken broth

¼ teaspoon freshly ground pepper

1 tablespoon chopped fresh basil or 1 teaspoon dried basil

NUTRIENT ANALYSIS FOR ONE SERVING

Calories from Fat 23%	**Calories from Carbs** 54%	**Total Fat** 2 g
Protein 4 g	**Carbohydrates** 10 g	**Saturated Fat** 0 g
Sodium 78 mg	**Fiber** 2 g	**Monounsaturated Fat** 1 g
Cholesterol 0 mg	**Sugars** 6 g	**Polyunsaturated Fat** 0 g

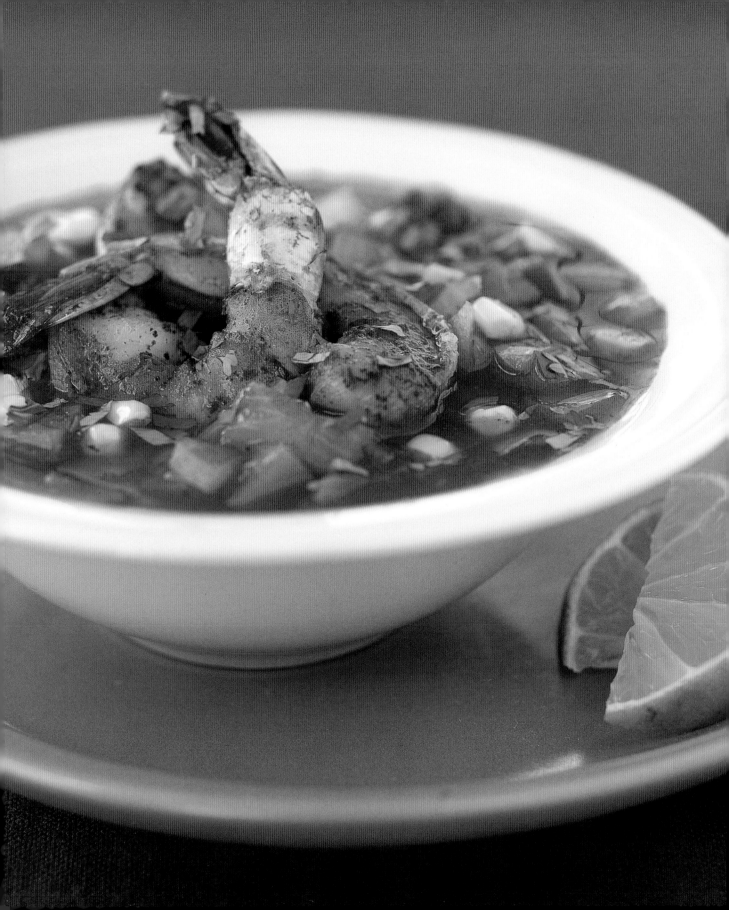

SHRIMP & SWEET CORN SOUP

CALORIES 105

DIABETIC EXCHANGES
| ½ starch | 0 fruit | 0 milk |
| 1½ vegetable | 1½ protein | ½ fat |

SERVES 6

This soup is a heart-healthy, low-fat version of chili, but with fresher flavors. Served with a salad and crusty whole-grain bread, it's substantial enough for a main dish. Or serve it as a first course for any meal with a Mexican theme.

In a large saucepan over medium-high heat, heat 1 teaspoon of the olive oil. Add the onion and bell pepper and sauté until softened, about 5 minutes. Add the garlic, 2 teaspoons of the chili powder, and 1 teaspoon of the cumin and cook for 1 minute. Add the broth and bring to a boil. Reduce the heat to medium-low and simmer, covered, stirring occasionally, until the vegetables are tender, about 5 minutes. Stir in the tomato, corn, and lime juice and simmer until the corn is tender, about 2 minutes.

While the soup is cooking, in a bowl, combine the remaining 1 teaspoon chili powder and ½ teaspoon cumin and stir to mix well. Add the shrimp and toss to coat.

In a nonstick frying pan over medium-high heat, heat the remaining 1 teaspoon olive oil. Add the shrimp and cook, stirring constantly, until the shrimp turn pink and are opaque throughout, about 3 minutes.

Ladle the soup into individual bowls and top each serving with the shrimp, dividing evenly. Sprinkle with the cilantro and serve with lime wedges, if desired.

2 teaspoons olive oil

1 yellow onion, chopped

1 red bell pepper (capsicum), chopped

2 cloves garlic, minced

3 teaspoons chili powder

1½ teaspoons ground cumin

3 cups (24 fl oz/750 ml) fat-free, no-salt-added chicken broth

1 tomato, chopped

½ cup (3 oz/90 g) fresh or frozen corn kernels

1 tablespoon fresh lime juice

½ lb (250 g) medium shrimp, peeled and deveined

¼ cup (½ oz/15 g) chopped fresh cilantro (fresh coriander) or parsley

Lime wedges for serving (optional)

NUTRIENT ANALYSIS FOR ONE SERVING

Calories from Fat 23%	**Calories from Carbs** 34%	**Total Fat** 3 g
Protein 12 g	**Carbohydrates** 9 g	**Saturated Fat** 0 g
Sodium 137 mg	**Fiber** 2 g	**Monounsaturated Fat** 1 g
Cholesterol 57 mg	**Sugars** 4 g	**Polyunsaturated Fat** 1 g

SESAME NOODLE SOUP

DIABETIC EXCHANGES

1 starch	0 fruit	0 milk
½ vegetable	1 protein	0 fat

SERVES 6

- 4 oz (125 g) whole-wheat (wholemeal) or 50-percent whole-wheat angel hair pasta
- 4½ cups (36 fl oz/1.1 l) fat-free, no-salt-added vegetable or chicken broth
- 1 tablespoon peeled and minced fresh ginger
- ⅛ teaspoon red pepper flakes
- 1 cup (5 oz/155 g) fresh snow peas (mangetouts), halved diagonally
- 4 oz (125 g) white mushrooms, brushed clean and sliced (about 1¼ cups)
- 4 cups (8 oz/250 g) chopped fresh spinach or baby spinach leaves
- ½ teaspoon dark sesame oil
- ¼ cup (¾ oz/20 g) thinly sliced green (spring) onions

Whenever you need comforting with a steaming bowl of noodle soup, try this gingery version. If shiitake mushrooms are available, substitute them for the white mushrooms to create a more pungent, fragrant soup.

Bring a large pot three-fourths full of water to a boil. Add the pasta and cook until al dente, about 7 minutes, or according to package directions. Drain the pasta thoroughly and set aside.

In a large saucepan, combine the broth, ginger, and red pepper flakes and bring to a boil over medium-high heat. Add the snow peas and mushrooms and cook, uncovered, until the vegetables are softened, about 1 minute. Add the spinach, sesame oil, and pasta and cook until the spinach wilts, about 30 seconds. Ladle the soup into individual bowls and sprinkle with the green onions.

NUTRIENT ANALYSIS FOR ONE SERVING

Calories from Fat 6%	**Calories from Carbs** 66%	**Total Fat** 1 g
Protein 7 g	**Carbohydrates** 17 g	**Saturated Fat** 0 g
Sodium 112 mg	**Fiber** 3 g	**Monounsaturated Fat** 0 g
Cholesterol 0 mg	**Sugars** 2 g	**Polyunsaturated Fat** 0 g

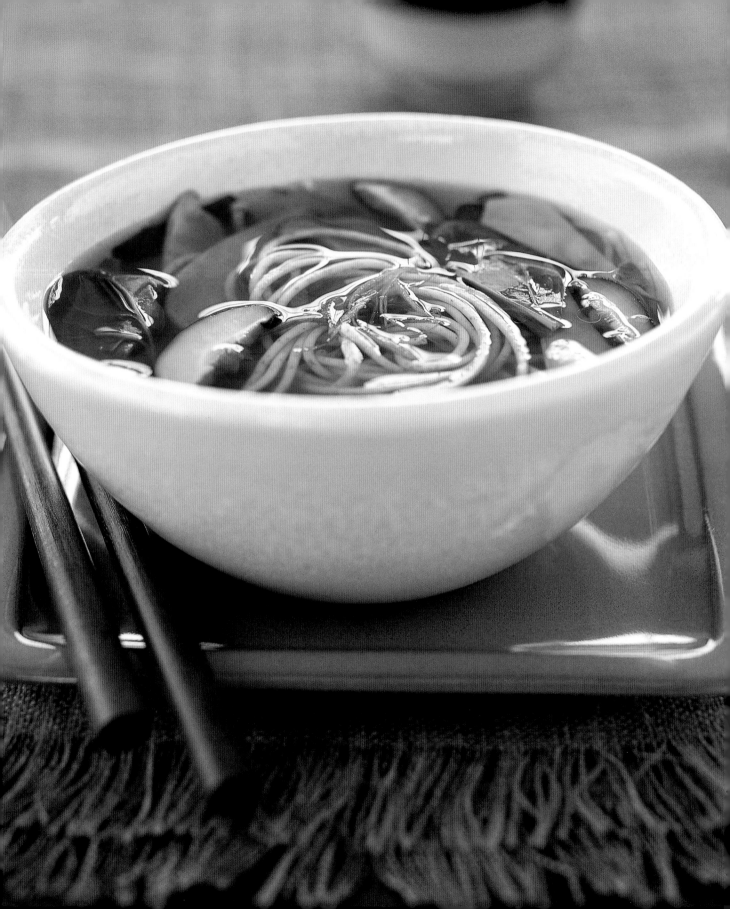

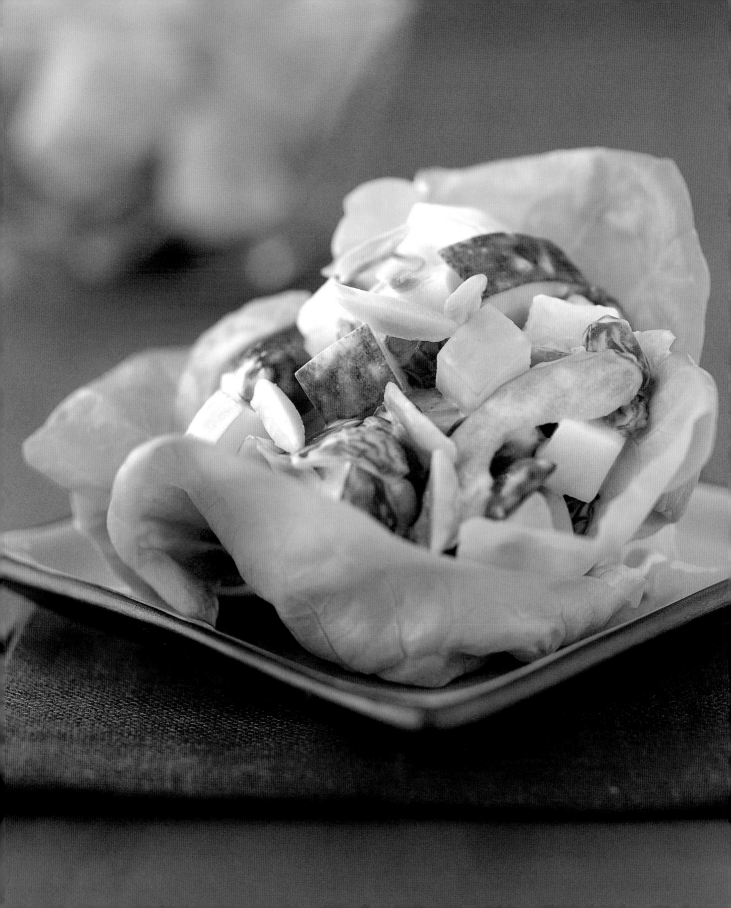

APPLE, RAISIN & ALMOND SALAD

DIABETIC EXCHANGES

0 starch	1½ fruit	0 milk
0 vegetable	2 protein	½ fat

SERVES 6   Kid-friendly recipe

Make an extra batch of this nutrient-dense salad for packing in lunches during the week. It stores well for up to 3 days in the refrigerator. For an elegant brunch, serve it with Vegetable & Goat Cheese Strata (page 82).

Put the almonds in a small, dry, nonstick frying pan over medium-low heat. Cook, stirring constantly, until lightly toasted, about 2 minutes. Transfer to a plate and set aside.

In a large bowl, combine the apples, celery, grapes, raisins, and yogurt and stir to mix well. To serve, place a lettuce leaf on each of 6 plates and divide the apple mixture evenly among the lettuce leaves. Sprinkle with the toasted almonds just before serving so the nuts remain crisp.

¼ cup (1 oz/30 g) sliced (flaked) almonds

2 Gala or McIntosh apples, halved, cored, and cut into ¾-inch (2-cm) pieces

2 Granny Smith apples, halved, cored, and cut into ¾-inch (2-cm) pieces

1 celery stalk, thinly sliced

½ cup (3 oz/90 g) red seedless grapes, cut in half

¼ cup (1½ oz/45 g) golden raisins

½ cup (4 oz/125 g) low-fat yogurt

6 Bibb lettuce leaves

NUTRIENT ANALYSIS FOR ONE SERVING

Calories from Fat 18%	**Calories from Carbs** 73%	**Total Fat** 2 g
Protein 3 g	**Carbohydrates** 21 g	**Saturated Fat** 0 g
Sodium 22 mg	**Fiber** 3 g	**Monounsaturated Fat** 1 g
Cholesterol 1 mg	**Sugars** 17 g	**Polyunsaturated Fat** 0 g

54

TOMATO & CUCUMBER SALAD WITH MINT PESTO

DIABETIC EXCHANGES

0 starch	0 fruit	0 milk
1 vegetable	0 protein	0 fat

SERVES 4

½ cup (½ oz/15 g) loosely packed fresh mint leaves

½ cup (½ oz/15 g) loosely packed fresh parsley leaves

1 tablespoon slivered almonds

1 tablespoon grated Parmesan cheese

1 clove garlic, chopped

1 teaspoon grated lemon zest

1 tablespoon fresh lemon juice

2 tablespoons fat-free, no-salt-added vegetable or chicken broth

3 tomatoes, sliced

1 English (hothouse) cucumber, peeled and sliced on the diagonal

Use the bounty of summer tomatoes and cucumbers to make this refreshing salad. For even more flavor and a prettier presentation, use different colors and varieties of tomatoes. The mint pesto is perfect for grilled salmon and lamb chops, too.

In a food processor or blender, combine the mint, parsley, almonds, Parmesan, and garlic and pulse until the herbs are coarsely chopped. Add the lemon zest and juice and broth and process until well blended.

Arrange the tomato and cucumber slices on individual plates and top with the pesto. Serve immediately.

NUTRIENT ANALYSIS FOR ONE SERVING

Calories from Fat 27%	**Calories from Carbs** 54%	**Total Fat** 2 g
Protein 3 g	**Carbohydrates** 8 g	**Saturated Fat** 0 g
Sodium 44 mg	**Fiber** 3 g	**Monounsaturated Fat** 1 g
Cholesterol 1 mg	**Sugars** 4 g	**Polyunsaturated Fat** 0 g

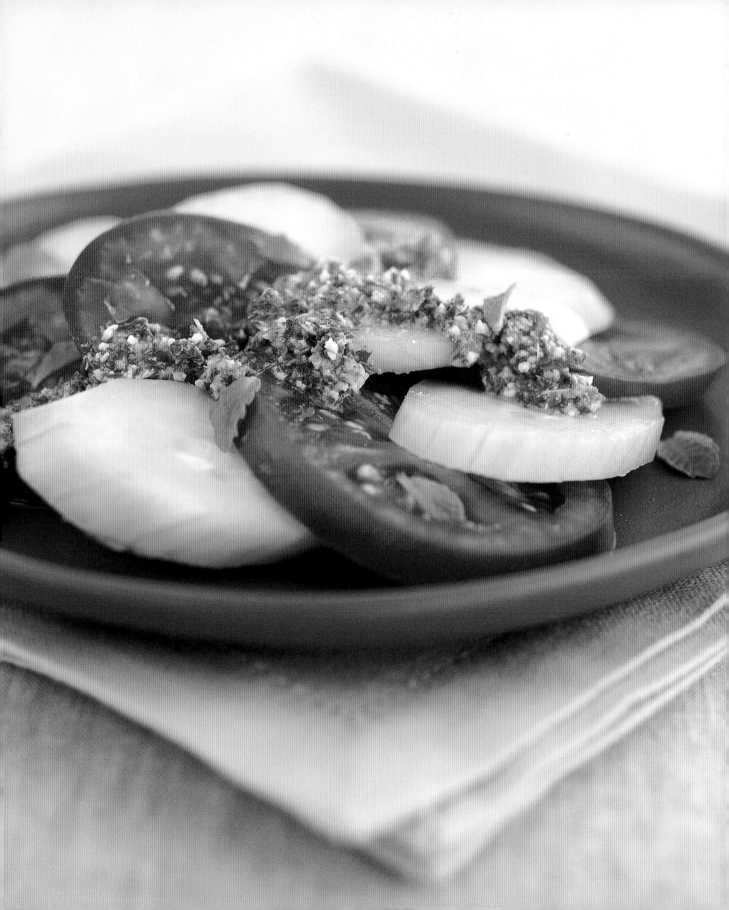

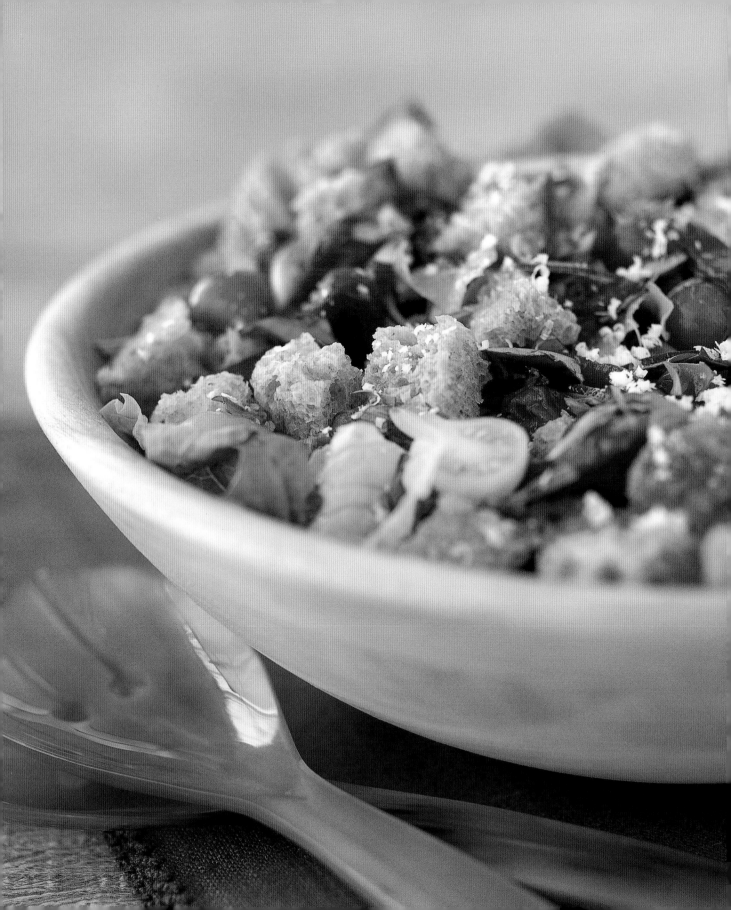

BREAD SALAD WITH ROASTED RED PEPPERS

CALORIES **103**

SERVES 6

DIABETIC EXCHANGES

| ½ starch | 0 fruit | 0 milk |
| 1 vegetable | ½ protein | ½ fat |

Vegetable broth is a light base for the dressing in this salad, letting the taste of the tomatoes, roasted peppers, and herbs shine through. When using fresh parsley and basil, try keeping the leaves whole to add texture and big bursts of vibrant flavor.

Preheat the oven to 350°F (180°C). Place the bread cubes in a single layer in a shallow roasting pan or rimmed baking sheet. Bake, stirring once, until lightly toasted, about 8 minutes. Let cool to room temperature.

While the bread is toasting, in a large bowl, combine the broth, vinegar, olive oil, and ground pepper and stir to mix well. Add the roasted red peppers, tomatoes, onion, basil, and parsley, if using. Toss to coat. Add the toasted bread cubes and the lettuce and toss just until the ingredients are evenly distributed. Divide the salad among individual plates, top with the Parmesan, and serve immediately.

4 oz (125 g) sturdy whole-grain bread, cut into ½-inch (12-mm) cubes (about 2½ cups)

¼ cup (2 fl oz/60 ml) fat-free, no-salt-added vegetable or chicken broth

2 tablespoons balsamic vinegar

2 teaspoons olive oil

¼ teaspoon freshly ground pepper

½ cup (4 oz/125 g) roasted red peppers from a jar, drained and cut into thin strips

1 cup (6 oz/185 g) cherry tomatoes, halved

¼ cup (1 oz/30 g) thinly sliced red onion

¼ cup (½ oz/15 g) chopped fresh basil or 1 teaspoon dried basil

¼ cup (½ oz/15 g) chopped fresh parsley (optional)

4 cups (8 oz/250 g) torn romaine lettuce

¼ cup (1 oz/30 g) finely shredded Parmesan cheese

NUTRIENT ANALYSIS FOR ONE SERVING

Calories from Fat 29%	**Calories from Carbs** 57%	**Total Fat** 3 g
Protein 4 g	**Carbohydrates** 17 g	**Saturated Fat** 1 g
Sodium 192 mg	**Fiber** 5 g	**Monounsaturated Fat** 2 g
Cholesterol 3 mg	**Sugars** 4 g	**Polyunsaturated Fat** 0 g

SESAME SLAW

SERVES 4

2 teaspoons rice wine vinegar or white wine vinegar

1 tablespoon low-sodium soy sauce

1 tablespoon peeled and minced fresh ginger

1 teaspoon dark sesame oil

2 cups (6 oz/185 g) thinly sliced red cabbage

2 cups (6 oz/185 g) thinly sliced green cabbage

1 carrot, peeled and coarsely grated

2 tablespoons thinly sliced green (spring) onion

Dark sesame oil, found in the Asian foods section of most supermarkets, is a must-have pantry staple if you're watching fat and calories. As this simple slaw recipe shows, you need only a teaspoon of this aromatic oil to flavor an entire dish.

In a large bowl, combine the vinegar, soy sauce, ginger, and sesame oil and stir to combine. Add the cabbages, carrot, and green onion and toss gently to combine. Serve immediately or cover and refrigerate overnight.

NUTRIENT ANALYSIS FOR ONE SERVING

Calories from Fat 29%	Calories from Carbs 58%	Total Fat 1 g
Protein 1 g	Carbohydrates 6 g	Saturated Fat 0 g
Sodium 122 mg	Fiber 2 g	Monounsaturated Fat 0 g
Cholesterol 0 mg	Sugars 2 g	Polyunsaturated Fat 1 g

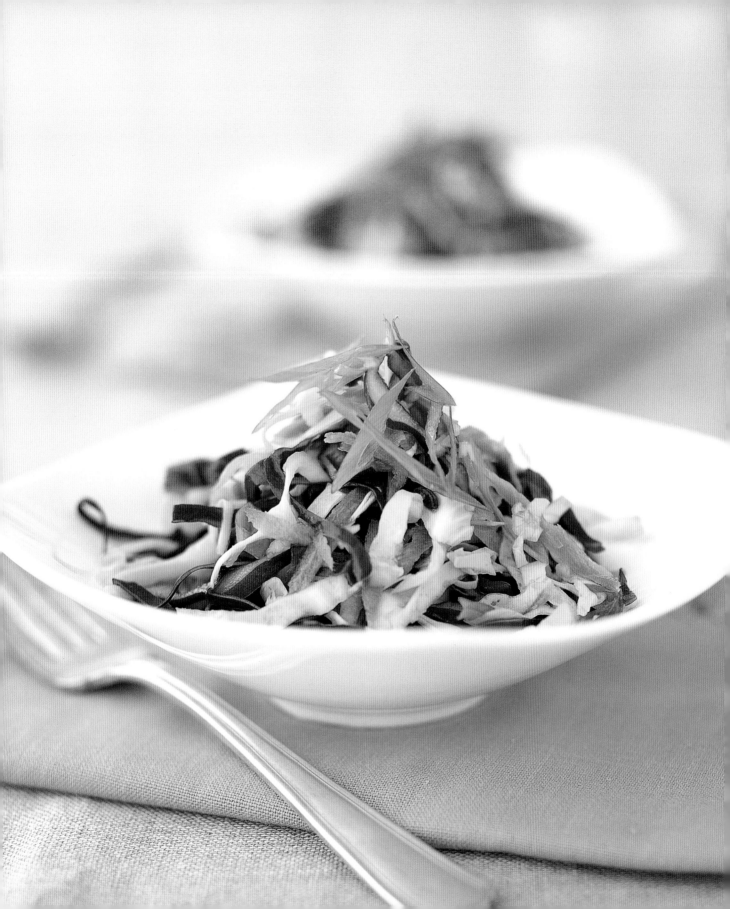

118

CALORIES

DIABETIC EXCHANGES

1 starch	0 fruit	0 milk
½ vegetable	0 protein	½ fat

BULGUR SALAD WITH FENNEL & SPINACH

SERVES 6

1 cup (6 oz/185 g) bulgur

1½ cups (12 fl oz/375 ml)
   boiling water

1 teaspoon grated lemon zest

3 tablespoons fresh lemon juice

3 tablespoons fat-free,
   no-salt-added vegetable or
   chicken broth

1 tablespoon olive oil

¼ teaspoon freshly ground pepper

1 large fennel bulb, about
   1 lb (500 g)

3 cups (6 oz/185 g) chopped fresh
   spinach or baby spinach leaves

If fennel is not available, use a peeled and thinly sliced cucumber and a sliced red bell pepper (capsicum) for flavor and crunch. When making the salad a day ahead, combine everything except the spinach, and stir it in just before serving.

Place the bulgur in a large, heatproof bowl and add the boiling water. Cover the bowl and let stand until the bulgur is tender and the water is completely absorbed, about 25 minutes.

While the bulgur is soaking, in a large bowl, combine the lemon zest and juice, broth, olive oil, and pepper and stir well to combine. Add the bulgur and toss gently until well combined. Let cool to room temperature.

Trim the tough outer stalks from the fennel bulb and cut in half lengthwise. Cut away and discard the core and cut the bulb into thin slices. Add the fennel and the spinach to the bowl with the bulgur mixture and toss just until the ingredients are evenly distributed. Serve at room temperature.

NUTRIENT ANALYSIS FOR ONE SERVING

Calories from Fat 19%	**Calories from Carbs** 69%	**Total Fat** 3 g
Protein 4 g	**Carbohydrates** 22 g	**Saturated Fat** 0 g
Sodium 42 mg	**Fiber** 6 g	**Monounsaturated Fat** 2 g
Cholesterol 0 mg	**Sugars** 0 g	**Polyunsaturated Fat** 0 g

AVOCADO, CORN & BLACK BEAN SALAD

SERVES 4

DIABETIC EXCHANGES

1 starch	0 fruit	0 milk
1 vegetable	½ protein	1 fat

Haas avocados, with their pebbly, dark green skin, have a creamier texture and richer flavor than the smooth-skinned varieties. You can assemble this salad and refrigerate it up to one day ahead; don't dress the romaine until ready to serve.

In a large bowl, combine the lime zest and juice, broth, olive oil, cumin, and pepper and stir to combine. Set the dressing aside.

In another bowl, combine the cucumber, tomatoes, corn, beans, avocado, and onion. Spoon 3 tablespoons of the dressing over the vegetables and toss to coat.

Add the lettuce to the bowl with the remaining dressing and toss gently to coat. Divide the lettuce among individual plates. Divide the bean mixture among the lettuce-lined plates and serve immediately.

½ teaspoon grated lime zest

2 tablespoons fresh lime juice

2 tablespoons fat-free, no-salt-added vegetable or chicken broth

1 teaspoon olive oil

¼ teaspoon ground cumin

¼ teaspoon freshly ground pepper

1 small cucumber, peeled, seeded, and chopped

2 plum (Roma) tomatoes, chopped

1 cup (6 oz/185 g) fresh corn kernels

1 cup (7 oz/220 g) canned no-salt-added black beans, rinsed and drained

½ cup (2½ oz/75 g) diced avocado

2 tablespoons minced red onion

4 cups (8 oz/250 g) thinly sliced romaine lettuce

NUTRIENT ANALYSIS FOR ONE SERVING

Calories from Fat 26%	**Calories from Carbs** 59%	**Total Fat** 5 g
Protein 6 g	**Carbohydrates** 24 g	**Saturated Fat** 1 g
Sodium 90 mg	**Fiber** 7 g	**Monounsaturated Fat** 3 g
Cholesterol 0 mg	**Sugars** 6 g	**Polyunsaturated Fat** 1 g

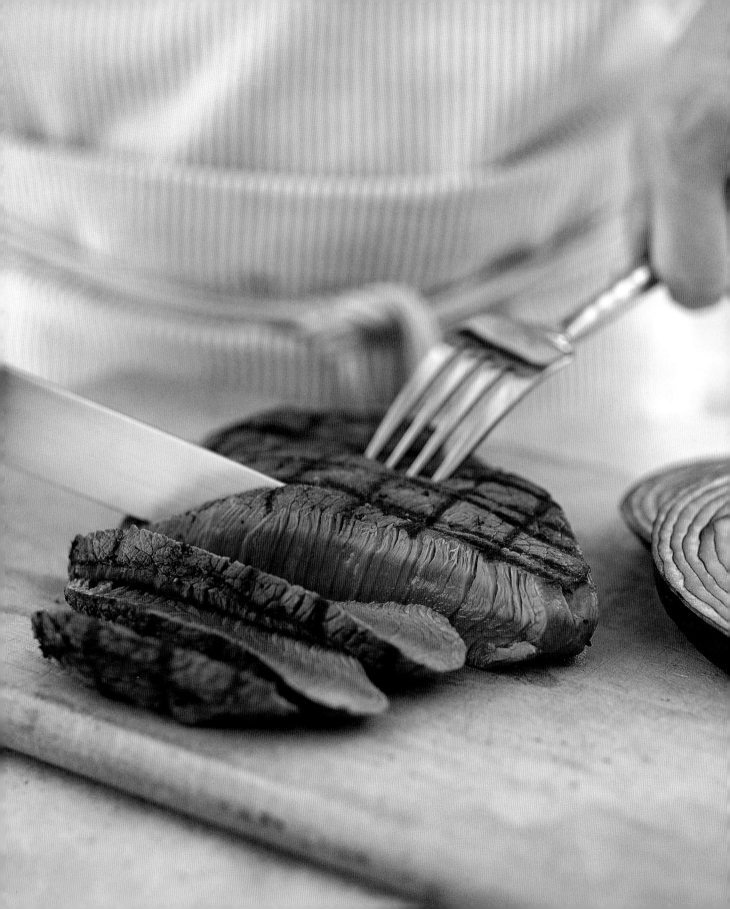

MAIN DISHES

122c ARTICHOKE & SPINACH FRITTATA, 88

170c VEGETABLE & GOAT CHEESE STRATA, 82

179c CHICKEN, VEGETABLE & BLACK BEAN CHILI, 64

183c PAN-SEARED TUNA WITH CUCUMBER-LEMON RELISH, 58

197c BRAISED HALIBUT WITH TOMATOES & THYME, 57

200c PORTOBELLOS STUFFED WITH VEGETABLES, 81

203c HERB-CRUSTED CHICKEN, 60

203c SNAPPER WITH SUMMER SQUASH & TOMATO, 54

203c RATATOUILLE PASTA, 80

206c GRILLED DIJON CHICKEN SALAD, 62

241c OVEN-POACHED SALMON, 59

242c VEGETABLE ENCHILADAS, 85

242c WHITE BEAN & BACON STEW, 92

249c ROASTED PORK LOIN WITH ACORN SQUASH, 71

253c BEEF TENDERLOIN WITH HERB SAUCE, 70

257c CURRIED TOFU & VEGETABLE STIR-FRY, 87

283c GRILLED STEAK, POTATOES & RED ONIONS, 68

286c PEANUT NOODLES WITH CHICKEN, 75

294c SPICED LENTILS, 91

298c CHEDDAR TURKEY BURGERS, 65

300c PORK CHOPS WITH APPLES & DATES, 67

307c PENNE WITH BROCCOLI & GARLIC, 76

340c BAKED MACARONI WITH VEGETABLES & CHEDDAR, 72

353c FETTUCCINE WITH SPRING VEGETABLES, 79

SNAPPER WITH SUMMER SQUASH & TOMATO

SERVES 4

2 teaspoons olive oil

4 snapper fillets, each about 5 oz (155 g) and ¾ inch (2 cm) thick

4 tablespoons (½ oz/15 g) chopped fresh basil or 2 teaspoons dried basil

½ teaspoon freshly ground pepper

1 clove garlic, minced

2 zucchini (courgettes), chopped

2 yellow crookneck squash, chopped

1 tomato, chopped

Fresh basil sprigs for garnish (optional)

Any mild-flavored white fish works well in this recipe. Try cod, tilapia, or striped bass if you can't find snapper. And you can substitute thyme, dill, or tarragon for the basil—almost any herb lends itself to this simple preparation.

Preheat the oven to 375°F (190°C). Select a shallow baking dish just large enough to hold the fillets in a single layer and coat the dish with 1 teaspoon of the olive oil.

Sprinkle the fillets on both sides with half of the basil and ¼ teaspoon of the pepper. Arrange the fillets in the prepared dish. Bake until the fillets are opaque throughout when tested in the center with the tip of a knife, 10–12 minutes.

While the fish is baking, in a nonstick sauté pan, heat the remaining 1 teaspoon olive oil over medium heat. Add the garlic and sauté for about 1 minute. Add the zucchini and yellow squash and sauté until almost tender, about 4 minutes. Stir in the tomato and cook, stirring constantly, until heated through, about 1 minute. Stir in the remaining basil and remaining ¼ teaspoon pepper. Divide the squash mixture evenly among individual plates. Top each serving with a fish fillet. Garnish with the fresh basil sprigs, if using.

NUTRIENT ANALYSIS FOR ONE SERVING

Calories from Fat 21%	**Calories from Carbs** 17%	**Total Fat** 5 g
Protein 32 g	**Carbohydrates** 9 g	**Saturated Fat** 1 g
Sodium 113 mg	**Fiber** 3 g	**Monounsaturated Fat** 2 g
Cholesterol 52 mg	**Sugars** 4 g	**Polyunsaturated Fat** 1 g

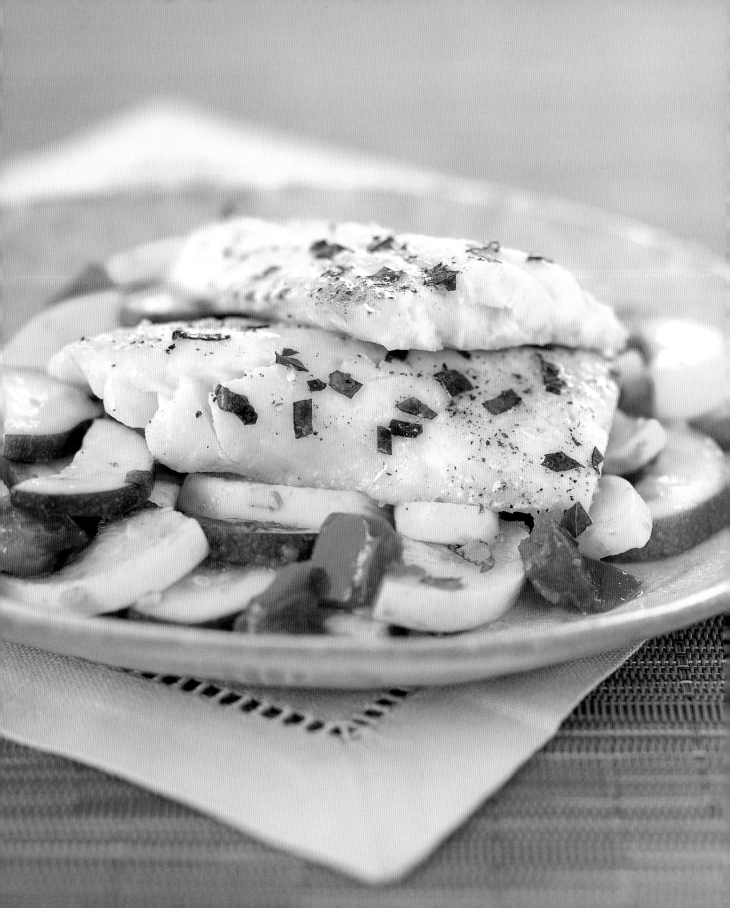

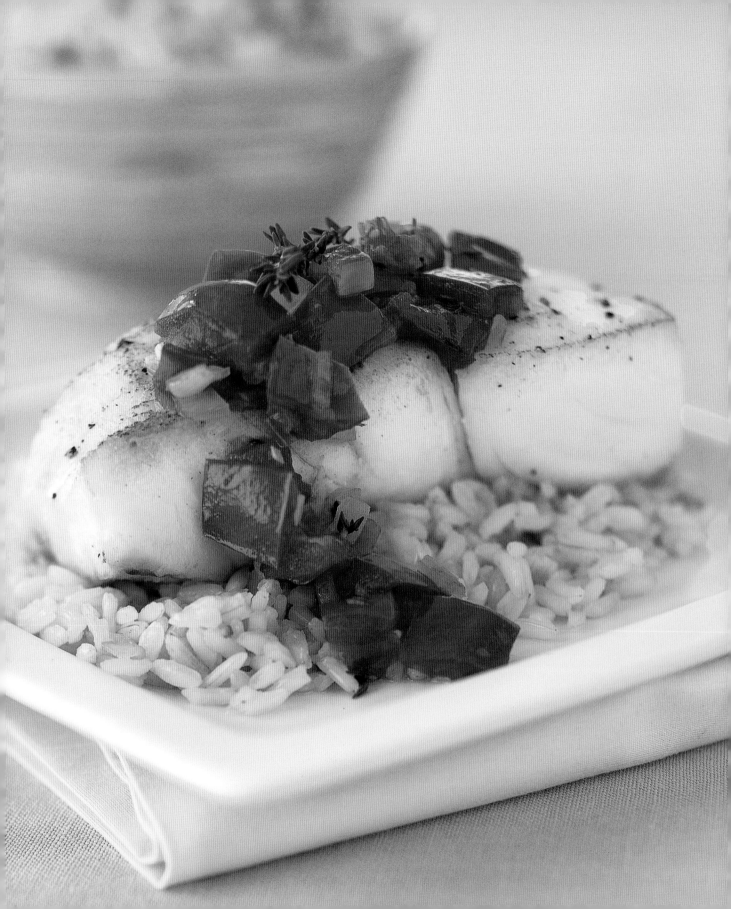

BRAISED HALIBUT WITH TOMATOES & THYME

SERVES 4

CALORIES 197

DIABETIC EXCHANGES

| 0 starch | 0 fruit | 0 milk |
| 1 vegetable | 4½ protein | 1 fat |

Get a heart-healthy dose of omega-6 fatty acids from the fish in this dish, and serve it on a bed of brown rice for extra fiber. If you use dried thyme, stir a few tablespoons of chopped fresh parsley into the sauce before serving for extra color and flavor.

In a large, nonstick frying pan, heat the olive oil over medium-high heat. Sprinkle the fillets with ¼ teaspoon of the pepper. Add the fish to the pan and cook, turning once, until lightly browned on both sides, about 1 minute per side. Transfer the fillets to a platter.

Add the shallots to the pan and sauté until they begin to soften, about 3 minutes. Add the garlic and sauté for 1 minute. Stir in the tomatoes, the broth, the remaining ¼ teaspoon pepper, and the thyme and bring to a boil. Return the fillets to the pan. Reduce the heat to low, cover, and simmer until the fillets are opaque throughout when tested in the center with the tip of a knife, 3–4 minutes.

To serve, place 1 fillet in each of 4 plates or shallow bowls. Top each with the tomato mixture and garnish with a sprig of thyme, if desired.

1 teaspoon olive oil

4 halibut fillets, each about 5 oz (155 g) and ¾ inch (2 cm) thick

½ teaspoon freshly ground pepper

3 shallots, diced

1 clove garlic, minced

2 large tomatoes, chopped

1 cup (8 fl oz/250 ml) fat-free, no-salt-added chicken broth

1 tablespoon chopped fresh thyme or 1 teaspoon dried thyme

Fresh thyme sprigs for garnish (optional)

NUTRIENT ANALYSIS FOR ONE SERVING

Calories from Fat 22%	**Calories from Carbs** 12%	**Total Fat** 5 g
Protein 32 g	**Carbohydrates** 6 g	**Saturated Fat** 1 g
Sodium 114 mg	**Fiber** 1 g	**Monounsaturated Fat** 2 g
Cholesterol 45 mg	**Sugars** 3 g	**Polyunsaturated Fat** 1 g

183

PAN-SEARED TUNA WITH CUCUMBER-LEMON RELISH

DIABETIC EXCHANGES

0 starch	0 fruit	0 milk
0 vegetable	5 protein	½ fat

SERVES 6

- 1 large lemon
- 1 large English cucumber, peeled, cut in half lengthwise, seeded, and sliced (about 2 cups)
- 1 green (spring) onion, including tender green parts, thinly sliced
- 2 tablespoons chopped fresh parsley
- 3 teaspoons olive oil
- 6 tuna steaks, each about 5 oz (155 g) and ½ inch (12 mm) thick
- ¼ teaspoon freshly ground pepper

A tangy, crunchy lemon-cucumber relish is the perfect match for rich tuna steaks. If you prefer more sweetness, use a Meyer lemon. For a meal that's simple but fancy enough for guests, serve it with Double Pea Sauté with Mint (page 108).

Grate the zest from the lemon (page 139) and place it in a bowl. Cut a thin slice from the top and bottom of the lemon, exposing the flesh. Stand the lemon upright and, using a sharp knife, thickly cut off the peel, following the contour of the fruit and removing all the white pith and membrane. Holding the lemon over the bowl containing the zest, carefully cut along both sides of each section to free it from the membrane. As you work, discard any seeds and let the sections fall into the bowl. Using two forks, break up the sections into small bits. Add the cucumber, green onion, parsley, and 2 teaspoons of the olive oil and toss to mix well. Set aside.

Heat a large, heavy-bottomed frying pan over medium heat. Add the remaining 1 teaspoon olive oil and tilt the pan to coat completely. Sprinkle the tuna steaks with the pepper. Add the tuna to the pan and cook, turning once, until the fish is opaque throughout and shows only a small amount of pink in the center when tested with the tip of a knife, about 1 minute per side. Transfer to individual plates and serve hot, topped with the relish.

NUTRIENT ANALYSIS FOR ONE SERVING

Calories from Fat 19%	**Calories from Carbs** 5%	**Total Fat** 4 g
Protein 34 g	**Carbohydrates** 2 g	**Saturated Fat** 1 g
Sodium 54 mg	**Fiber** 1 g	**Monounsaturated Fat** 2 g
Cholesterol 64 mg	**Sugars** 1 g	**Polyunsaturated Fat** 1 g

OVEN-POACHED SALMON

SERVES 4

To dress up fillets of good-for-the-heart salmon, experiment with different herbs; basil, oregano, and rosemary are good options. For a complete meal, serve the dish with whole-wheat (wholemeal) pasta and a salad of mixed greens.

Preheat the oven to 350°F (180°C).

In an ovenproof frying pan, heat the olive oil over medium heat. Add the onion and sauté until tender, about 5 minutes. Add the garlic and cook for 1 minute. Stir in the wine and broth and bring to a boil. Add the tomatoes and dill and stir to mix well. Place the salmon fillets in the pan on top of the tomatoes. Sprinkle the salmon with the pepper and lemon zest. Transfer to the oven, cover, and bake until the fish is opaque throughout when tested in the center with the tip of a knife, about 15 minutes.

To serve, place the fillets in individual shallow bowls and spoon the tomato mixture around the fish. Garnish with the dill sprigs, if desired.

2 teaspoons olive oil

1 yellow onion, halved lengthwise and thinly sliced crosswise

1 clove garlic, minced

½ cup (4 fl oz/125 ml) dry white wine or fat-free, no-salt-added chicken broth

½ cup (4 fl oz/125 ml) fat-free, no-salt-added chicken broth

2 tomatoes, chopped

2 tablespoons chopped fresh dill or 1 teaspoon dried dill

4 skinless salmon fillets, each about 5 oz (155 g) and ½ inch (12 mm) thick

¼ teaspoon freshly ground pepper

1 teaspoon grated lemon zest

Fresh dill sprigs for garnish (optional)

NUTRIENT ANALYSIS FOR ONE SERVING

Calories from Fat 28%	**Calories from Carbs** 13%	**Total Fat** 7 g
Protein 30 g	**Carbohydrates** 8 g	**Saturated Fat** 1 g
Sodium 118 mg	**Fiber** 2 g	**Monounsaturated Fat** 3 g
Cholesterol 74 mg	**Sugars** 4 g	**Polyunsaturated Fat** 2 g

HERB-CRUSTED CHICKEN

SERVES 4   Kid-friendly recipe

½ teaspoon olive oil

1 cup (2 oz/60 g) toasted whole-wheat (wholemeal) cereal flakes

⅓ cup (1½ oz/45 g) grated Parmesan cheese

2 tablespoons chopped fresh parsley (optional)

1 teaspoon dried oregano

1 egg

1 tablespoon water

4 skinless, boneless chicken breasts, about 4 oz (125 g) each

Crushed cereal flakes and Parmesan cheese make a crispy crust that keeps chicken moist and juicy. Serve the chicken with Green Beans with Leeks & Thyme (page 107) to add French flair to an all-American favorite.

Preheat the oven to 400°F (200°C). Lightly coat the bottom of a shallow roasting pan or rimmed baking sheet with the olive oil.

Place the cereal in a lock-top plastic bag and squeeze to crush the flakes into coarse crumbs. Place the crumbs in a shallow dish, add the Parmesan, parsley (if using), and oregano and stir to combine.

In another shallow dish, beat the egg and water together until combined. Dip each chicken breast in the egg mixture, then dredge in the crumb mixture, pressing to make the crumbs adhere. Place on the prepared pan and bake until the crust is lightly browned and the chicken is opaque throughout, 12–15 minutes. Serve immediately.

NUTRIENT ANALYSIS FOR ONE SERVING

Calories from Fat 25%	Calories from Carbs 13%	Total Fat 5 g
Protein 31 g	Carbohydrates 6 g	Saturated Fat 2 g
Sodium 226 mg	Fiber 1 g	Monounsaturated Fat 1 g
Cholesterol 120 mg	Sugars 1 g	Polyunsaturated Fat 1 g

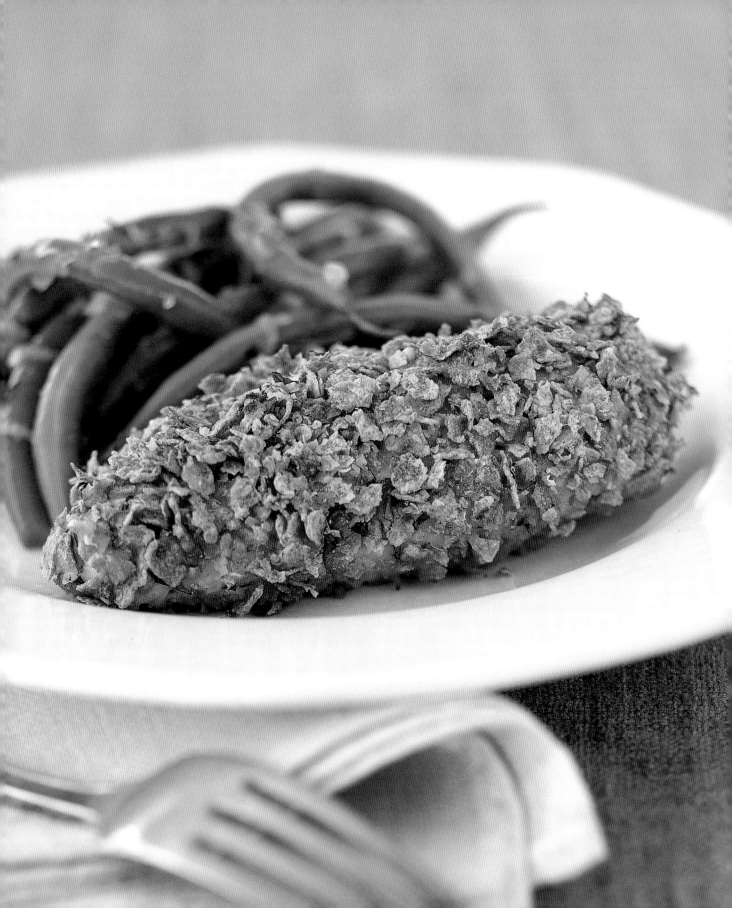

GRILLED DIJON CHICKEN SALAD

SERVES 4

- ½ lb (250 g) green beans, stems trimmed
- 1 clove garlic, minced
- 3 tablespoons fat-free, no-salt-added chicken broth
- 1 tablespoon olive oil
- 2 teaspoons plus 1 tablespoon Dijon mustard
- 1 teaspoon white wine vinegar
- ½ teaspoon freshly ground pepper
- 4 skinless, boneless chicken breasts, about 4 oz (125 g) each
- 4 cups (8 oz/250 g) torn romaine lettuce
- 2 cups (12 oz/375 g) cherry tomatoes, halved

Take care not to overcook skinless, boneless chicken breasts. A few minutes can mean the difference between moist and tender and overcooked and dry. Remove the breasts from the heat as soon as they are opaque throughout when cut into with a knife.

Prepare a fire in a charcoal grill or preheat a gas grill or oven broiler. Lightly coat the grill rack or broiler pan with olive oil cooking spray. Position the grill rack or broiler pan 4–6 inches (10–15 cm) from the heat source.

In a saucepan fitted with a steamer basket, bring 1 inch (2.5 cm) of water to a boil. Add the green beans, cover, and steam until tender, 4–5 minutes. Remove from the heat, drain, and rinse with cold water until the beans are cool. Drain thoroughly and set aside.

In a bowl, whisk together the garlic, broth, olive oil, 2 teaspoons of the mustard, the vinegar, and ¼ teaspoon of the pepper. Set the dressing aside.

Place the chicken in a shallow dish and sprinkle with the remaining ¼ teaspoon pepper. Brush with the remaining 1 tablespoon mustard to coat each breast completely. Grill or broil the chicken, turning once, until browned on both sides and opaque throughout, about 3 minutes per side.

In a large bowl, combine the lettuce and 1 tablespoon of the dressing. Toss to coat. Divide the lettuce evenly among individual plates. Thinly slice each chicken breast across the grain and arrange one sliced breast on top of the lettuce-lined plate. Arrange the green beans and tomatoes on top of each serving and drizzle each with some of the remaining dressing.

NUTRIENT ANALYSIS FOR ONE SERVING

Calories from Fat 23%	Calories from Carbs 20%	Total Fat 5 g
Protein 30 g	Carbohydrates 11 g	Saturated Fat 1 g
Sodium 243 mg	Fiber 4 g	Monounsaturated Fat 3 g
Cholesterol 66 mg	Sugars 3 g	Polyunsaturated Fat 1 g

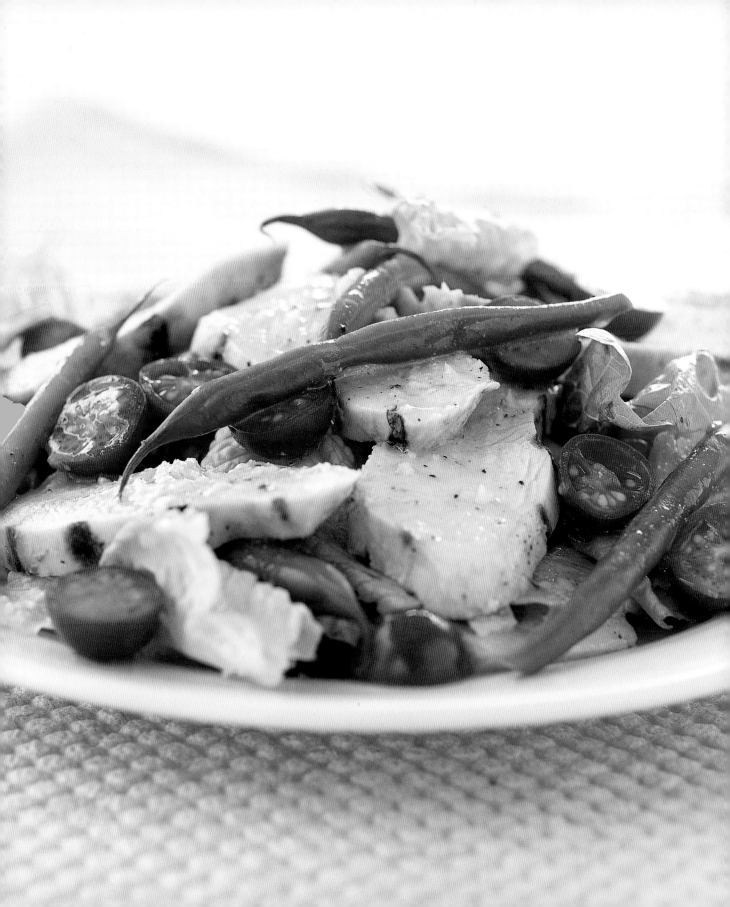

CHICKEN, VEGETABLE & BLACK BEAN CHILI

DIABETIC EXCHANGES

1 starch	0 fruit	0 milk
2 vegetable	2 protein	½ fat

SERVES 6

- 1 zucchini (courgette), cut into ½-inch (12-mm) chunks
- 1 yellow crookneck squash, cut into ½-inch (12-mm) chunks
- 2 teaspoons olive oil
- 8 oz (250 g) skinless, boneless chicken breast, cut into ½-inch (12-mm) cubes
- 1 yellow onion, chopped
- 1 green bell pepper (capsicum), chopped
- 1 clove garlic, minced
- 2 tablespoons chili powder
- 2 teaspoons ground cumin
- 2 cups (16 fl oz/500 ml) fat-free, no-salt-added chicken broth
- One 14-oz (440-g) can no-salt-added diced tomatoes
- One 15-oz (470-g) can no-salt-added black beans, rinsed and drained

Most beans are powerhouses of heart-healthy fiber, but when canned, they are often packed with added sodium. Read labels of canned beans carefully, choose brands that do not have added salt, and always rinse before using.

Preheat the oven to 450°F (230°C). Combine the squashes and 1 teaspoon of the olive oil in a shallow roasting pan or rimmed baking sheet and toss to coat. Roast, turning once, until the vegetables are tender and lightly browned, about 30 minutes.

While the vegetables are roasting, heat the remaining 1 teaspoon olive oil over medium heat in a large pot. Add the chicken and cook, stirring often, until opaque throughout, about 5 minutes. Add the onion, bell pepper, and garlic and cook, stirring often, until the vegetables are softened, about 5 minutes.

Stir in the chili powder and cumin and cook for 2 minutes longer. Add the broth, tomatoes, and beans and bring to a boil. Reduce the heat to medium-low and simmer, covered, until the vegetables are tender, 10–15 minutes. Stir in the roasted squashes and simmer for 5 minutes longer. Ladle into individual bowls and serve immediately.

NUTRIENT ANALYSIS FOR ONE SERVING

Calories from Fat 18%	**Calories from Carbs** 47%	**Total Fat** 4 g
Protein 16 g	**Carbohydrates** 22 g	**Saturated Fat** 1 g
Sodium 232 mg	**Fiber** 7 g	**Monounsaturated Fat** 1 g
Cholesterol 24 mg	**Sugars** 8 g	**Polyunsaturated Fat** 0 g

CHEDDAR TURKEY BURGERS

CALORIES 298

DIABETIC EXCHANGES

2 starch	0 fruit	0 milk
½ vegetable	3 protein	2 fat

SERVES 4

Kid-friendly recipe

With this low-fat, nutrient-rich recipe, you can put burgers back in family meals. These wonderfully juicy and flavorful turkey burgers will please both children and adults. Serve with Sweet Potato Oven Fries (page 96).

In a large bowl, combine the turkey, oats, egg white, onion, and pepper and mix with a large spoon or by hand until well blended. Shape the mixture into 4 patties about 4 inches (10 cm) in diameter.

Heat a large, nonstick frying pan over medium heat. Add the burgers, cover, and cook, turning occasionally, until no longer pink inside, 8–10 minutes. Sprinkle evenly with the cheese during the last minute of cooking.

Transfer the burgers to the buns, garnish with the tomato slices and lettuce leaves, and serve immediately.

¾ lb lean ground turkey

1 cup (3 oz/90 g) old-fashioned rolled oats

1 egg white

2 tablespoons grated yellow onion

¼ teaspoon freshly ground pepper

¼ cup (1 oz/30 g) finely shredded reduced-fat sharp Cheddar cheese

4 small whole-grain buns, split and toasted

4 tomato slices

4 lettuce leaves

NUTRIENT ANALYSIS FOR ONE SERVING

Calories from Fat 30%	**Calories from Carbs** 40%	**Total Fat** 10 g
Protein 23 g	**Carbohydrates** 30 g	**Saturated Fat** 3 g
Sodium 314 mg	**Fiber** 5 g	**Monounsaturated Fat** 4 g
Cholesterol 69 mg	**Sugars** 4 g	**Polyunsaturated Fat** 3 g

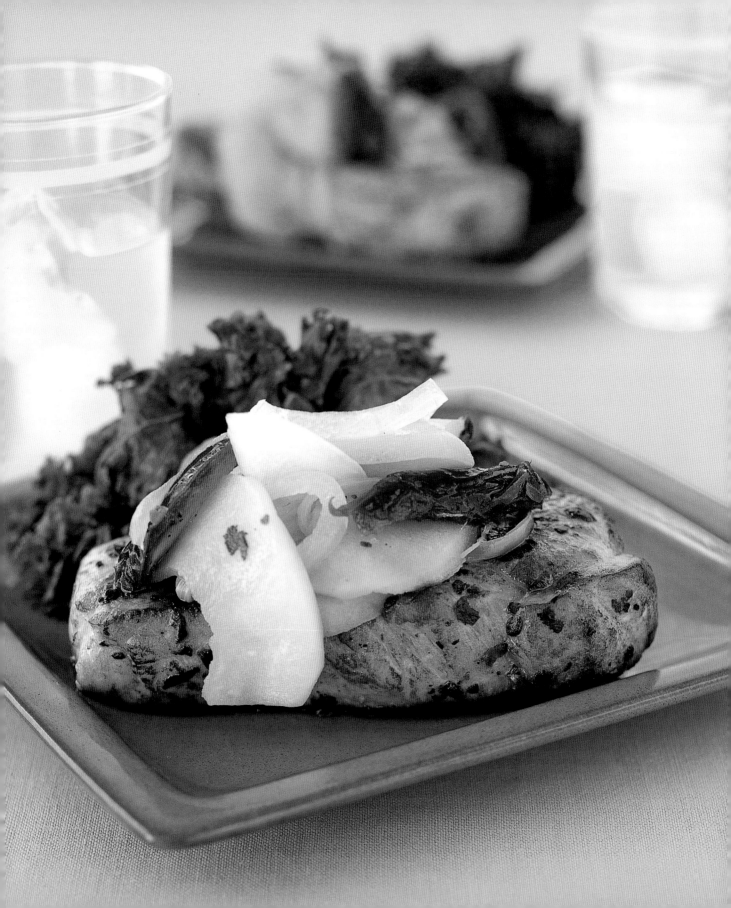

PORK CHOPS WITH APPLES & DATES

DIABETIC EXCHANGES

0 starch	2 fruit	0 milk
0 vegetable	3½ protein	1½ fat

SERVES 4

Discover the complex flavor and natural sweetness that dates lend to this easy recipe. For more vitamins and minerals, serve this hearty autumnal dish with steamed kale or mustard greens. Center-cut pork loin chops are quite lean and very easy to cook.

Sprinkle the pork chops with 1 tablespoon of the sage and the pepper. In a large, nonstick frying pan, heat 1 teaspoon of the olive oil over medium-high heat. Add the pork chops and cook, turning once, until the chops are opaque throughout, about 4 minutes on each side. Transfer to a platter and cover to keep warm.

Add the remaining 1 teaspoon olive oil to the pan. Add the onion and apples and cook, stirring often, until softened, about 5 minutes. Stir in the broth, vinegar, dates, and the remaining 2 teaspoons sage and cook, stirring constantly, until most of the liquid is absorbed, about 2 minutes longer.

To serve, place 1 chop on each of 4 plates. Top each serving evenly with the apple mixture and serve immediately.

4 boneless center-cut pork loin chops, 4 oz (125 g) each, trimmed of visible fat

1 tablespoon plus 2 teaspoons dried sage leaves

½ teaspoon freshly ground pepper

2 teaspoons olive oil

1 yellow onion, halved lengthwise and thinly sliced crosswise

2 Granny Smith apples, halved, cored, and sliced

½ cup (4 fl oz/125 ml) fat-free, no-salt-added chicken broth

2 teaspoons cider vinegar

½ cup (6 oz/185 g) dried dates, quartered

NUTRIENT ANALYSIS FOR ONE SERVING

Calories from Fat 27%	**Calories from Carbs** 41%	**Total Fat** 9 g
Protein 25 g	**Carbohydrates** 31 g	**Saturated Fat** 3 g
Sodium 67 mg	**Fiber** 4 g	**Monounsaturated Fat** 5 g
Cholesterol 67 mg	**Sugars** 24 g	**Polyunsaturated Fat** 1 g

GRILLED STEAK, POTATOES & RED ONIONS

SERVES 4

- 1 lb (500 g) small red or white potatoes, about 1-inch (2.5-cm) diameter
- 1 tablespoon red wine vinegar
- 1 teaspoon olive oil
- 1 tablespoon chopped fresh thyme or 1½ teaspoons dried thyme
- 1 lb (500 g) beef top sirloin steak, about 1 inch (2.5 cm) thick, trimmed of visible fat
- 2 red onions, cut crosswise into ½-inch (12-mm) slices
- ½ teaspoon freshly ground pepper
- Fresh thyme sprigs for garnish (optional)

A crisp green salad is all you need to complete this meat-and-potatoes meal. Top sirloin, top round, and flank steak are the best of the lean cuts of beef for grilling. They are all quick to cook, too, so a nutrient-rich dinner can be ready in minutes.

In a saucepan fitted with a steamer basket, bring 1 inch (2.5 cm) of water to a boil. Add the potatoes, cover, and steam until tender, about 10 minutes. Let cool slightly and cut each potato in half. While the potatoes are steaming, in a large bowl, whisk together the vinegar, olive oil, and thyme.

Prepare a fire in a charcoal grill or preheat a gas grill or oven broiler. Lightly coat the grill rack or broiler pan with olive oil cooking spray. Position the grill rack or broiler pan 4–6 inches (10–15 cm) from the heat source. Sprinkle the steak, potatoes, and onion slices with the pepper. Place the steak and onions on the grill rack or broiler pan. Grill or broil, turning once, until the onions are lightly browned and the steak is medium rare, about 4 minutes on each side. Cut into the steak to check for doneness.

Transfer the onions to the bowl with the vinegar mixture. Transfer the steak to a carving board and let rest for 5 minutes. Meanwhile, grill or broil the potatoes, turning once, until lightly browned, about 2 minutes on each side. Place the potatoes in the bowl with the onions and toss to combine. Cut the steak across the grain into thin slices.

To serve, divide the onions and potatoes among individual plates. Top with the sliced steak and serve hot. Garnish with the thyme sprigs, if desired.

NUTRIENT ANALYSIS FOR ONE SERVING

Calories from Fat 30%	**Calories from Carbs** 37%	**Total Fat** 9 g
Protein 23 g	**Carbohydrates** 25 g	**Saturated Fat** 3 g
Sodium 69 mg	**Fiber** 3 g	**Monounsaturated Fat** 4 g
Cholesterol 55 mg	**Sugars** 5 g	**Polyunsaturated Fat** 1 g

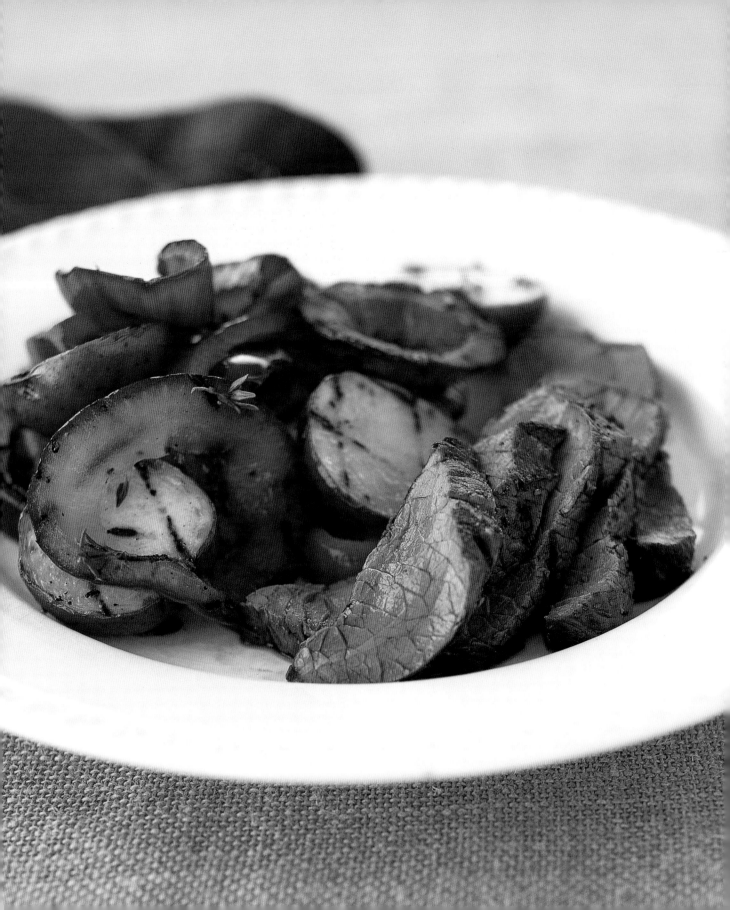

253

BEEF TENDERLOIN WITH HERB SAUCE

SERVES 4

2 long russet potatoes, about 1 lb (500 g) total weight, scrubbed and cut into ⅜-inch (1-cm) slices

2 teaspoons olive oil

¾ teaspoon freshly ground pepper

⅓ cup (⅓ oz/10 g) fresh parsley leaves

⅓ cup (⅓ oz/10 g) fresh mint leaves

⅓ cup (⅓ oz/10 g) fresh cilantro (fresh coriander) leaves

1 tablespoon minced green (spring) onion

2 cloves garlic, minced

⅓ cup (3 fl oz/80 ml) fat-free, no-salt-added chicken broth

2 tablespoons red wine vinegar

⅛ teaspoon red pepper flakes

4 beef tenderloin steaks, each about 4 oz (125 g) and 1 inch (2.5 cm) thick, trimmed of visible fat

The sauce for this dish is an adaptation of *chimichurri,* which Argentineans use to enhance the flavor of grilled meats. Tenderloin steaks, though pricey, work well here—they're exceptionally lean and tender, and they cook in minutes.

Preheat the oven to 400°F (200°C).

Place the potato slices in a large roasting pan or rimmed baking sheet. Drizzle with 1 teaspoon of the olive oil and sprinkle with ¼ teaspoon of the pepper. Toss to coat and arrange the potatoes in a single layer. Bake, turning once, until the potatoes are tender and lightly browned, about 25 minutes.

Meanwhile, in a blender, combine the parsley, mint, cilantro, green onion, garlic, broth, vinegar, the remaining 1 teaspoon olive oil, and the red pepper flakes. Process until the herbs are finely chopped. Set aside.

Heat a heavy-bottomed frying pan over medium heat. Sprinkle the steaks with the remaining ½ teaspoon black pepper. Place the steaks in the pan and cook, turning once, to the desired doneness, for about 2 minutes on each side for medium-rare. Cut into the steaks to check for doneness.

To serve, divide the steaks and potatoes among individual plates. Drizzle the steaks and potatoes with the herb sauce and serve immediately.

NUTRIENT ANALYSIS FOR ONE SERVING

Calories from Fat 28%	Calories from Carbs 32%	Total Fat 8 g
Protein 25 g	Carbohydrates 20 g	Saturated Fat 2 g
Sodium 69 mg	Fiber 3 g	Monounsaturated Fat 4 g
Cholesterol 52 mg	Sugars 1 g	Polyunsaturated Fat 0 g

ROASTED PORK LOIN WITH ACORN SQUASH

CALORIES 249

DIABETIC EXCHANGES
0 starch	0 fruit	0 milk
3½ vegetable	3½ protein	1 fat

SERVES 4

Pork tenderloin is juicy and succulent—as long as it's not overcooked. Take the meat out of the oven when it still has a slight blush of pink in the center. The tenderloin will continue to cook during the 5 minutes it rests before you slice it.

Preheat the oven to 400°F (200°C).

Cut the squash in half vertically, remove the seeds, and cut each half into 4 wedges, leaving the peel intact.

Place the squash in a large, shallow roasting pan or rimmed baking sheet. Drizzle with the olive oil and turn to coat. Sprinkle with half of the rosemary.

Place the pork in the pan and sprinkle with the pepper and the remaining rosemary. Roast, turning the squash slices and the pork once, until the squash is tender and the pork is firm to the touch and slightly pink inside, or until an instant-read thermometer inserted into the thickest part reads 160°F (70°C), 25–30 minutes. Let stand for 5 minutes.

To serve, divide the squash wedges among 4 plates. Slice the pork tenderloin crosswise into 16 slices and divide among the plates. Serve immediately.

1 acorn squash, about 2 lb (1 kg)

2 teaspoons olive oil

4 tablespoons chopped fresh rosemary or 4 teaspoons dried crumbled rosemary

1 pork tenderloin, about 1 lb, (500 g) trimmed of visible fat

½ teaspoon freshly ground pepper

NUTRIENT ANALYSIS FOR ONE SERVING

Calories from Fat 23%	**Calories from Carbs** 37%	**Total Fat** 6 g
Protein 26 g	**Carbohydrates** 24 g	**Saturated Fat** 2 g
Sodium 64 mg	**Fiber** 4 g	**Monounsaturated Fat** 4 g
Cholesterol 74 mg	**Sugars** 5 g	**Polyunsaturated Fat** 1 g

BAKED MACARONI WITH VEGETABLES & CHEDDAR

SERVES 4

Kid-friendly recipe

8 oz (250 g) whole-wheat (wholemeal) or 50-percent whole-wheat macaroni or other dried pasta

2 carrots, peeled and sliced

3 cups (6 oz/185 g) broccoli florets

1 tablespoon olive oil

1 tablespoon all-purpose (plain) flour

1½ cups (12 fl oz/375 ml) 1-percent milk

¾ cup (3 oz/ 90 g) shredded reduced-fat sharp Cheddar cheese

¼ teaspoon freshly ground pepper

This dish is comfort food at its healthiest. Be sure to use sharp Cheddar to get the most flavor from a small amount of cheese. Cook the vegetables along with the pasta to make preparing this weeknight favorite faster and even easier.

Preheat the oven to 350°F (180°C). Lightly coat an 11-by-7-inch (28-by18-cm) baking dish with olive oil cooking spray.

Bring a saucepan three-fourths full of water to a boil. Add the pasta and cook for 5 minutes. Stir in the carrots and cook for 3 minutes longer. Add the broccoli and cook for 2 minutes longer. Drain thoroughly and set aside.

While the pasta and vegetables are cooking, heat the olive oil in a large saucepan over medium heat. Add the flour and cook, stirring constantly, for 1 minute. Slowly add the milk, whisking constantly. Cook, whisking often, until the mixture comes to a boil and thickens slightly, about 5 minutes. Remove from the heat and add all but 2 tablespoons of the cheese, whisking until the cheese is melted. Add the pasta and vegetables to the cheese sauce and toss gently. Add the pepper and stir to mix well.

Spoon the mixture into the prepared dish. Sprinkle the top with the remaining 2 tablespoons cheese. Bake, uncovered, until the casserole is bubbly and the cheese is melted, about 15 minutes. Let stand for 5 minutes before serving.

NUTRIENT ANALYSIS FOR ONE SERVING

Calories from Fat 18%	**Calories from Carbs** 62%	**Total Fat** 7 g
Protein 19 g	**Carbohydrates** 55 g	**Saturated Fat** 2 g
Sodium 210 mg	**Fiber** 7 g	**Monounsaturated Fat** 4 g
Cholesterol 9 mg	**Sugars** 6 g	**Polyunsaturated Fat** 1 g

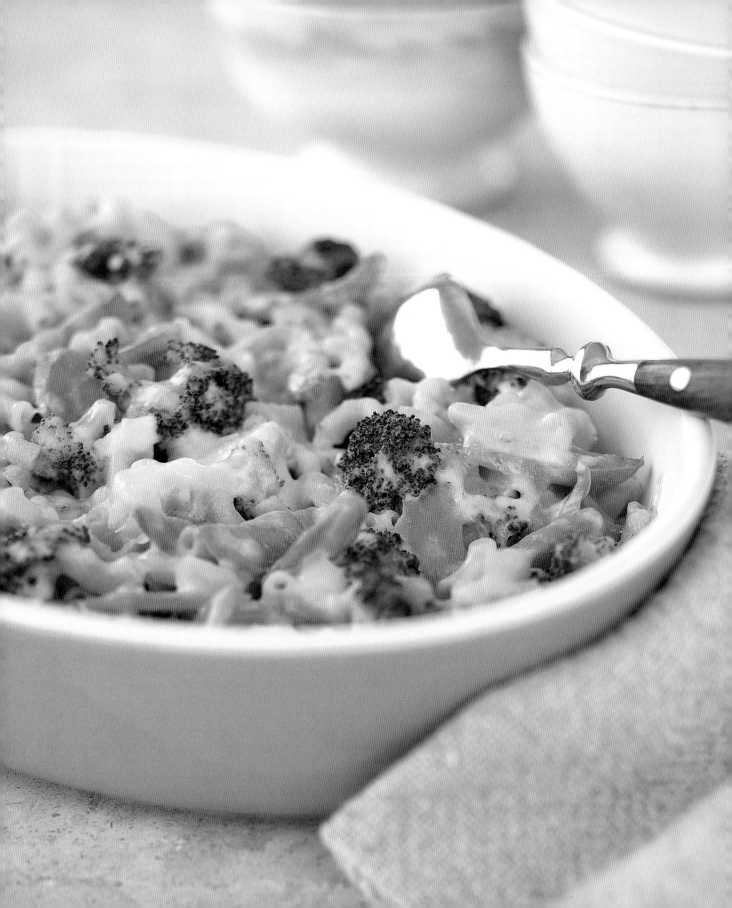

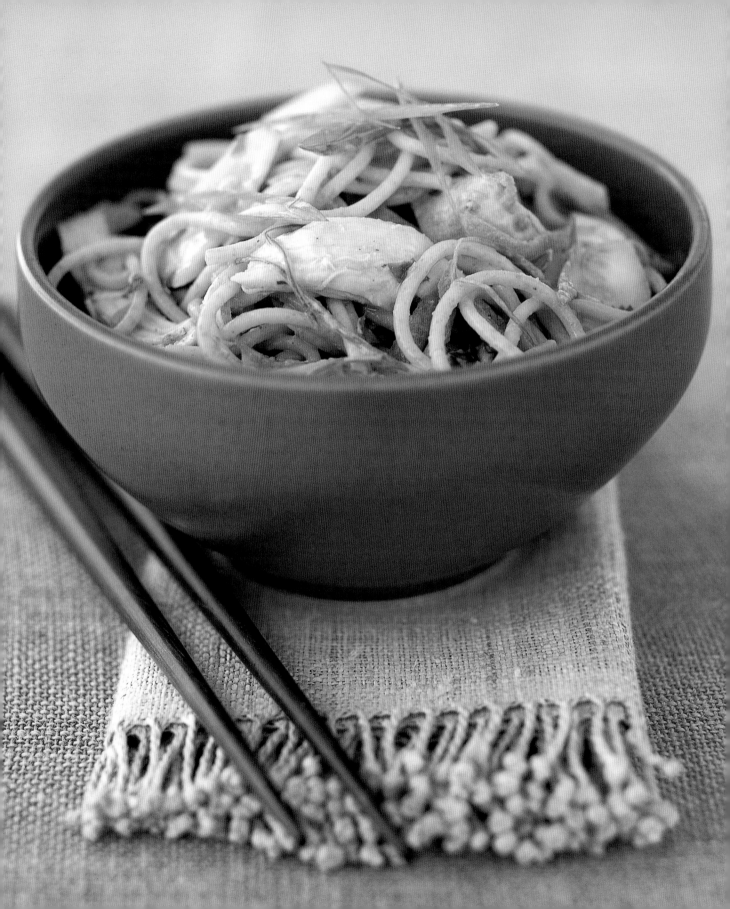

PEANUT NOODLES WITH CHICKEN

SERVES 6

Kid-friendly recipe

CALORIES 286

DIABETIC EXCHANGES

2 starch	0 fruit	0 milk
½ vegetable	3 protein	1 fat

To make the dressing for this salad, use natural peanut butter with no added sugars or salt. When made ahead, the pasta absorbs the dressing; if the noodles seem dry, stir in a few tablespoons of broth or water before serving.

In a large saucepan, combine the broth and chicken. Bring to a boil over high heat. Reduce the heat to low, cover, and simmer until the chicken is opaque throughout, 8–10 minutes. Transfer the chicken to a plate and let cool slightly. Discard the broth.

While the chicken is cooking, bring a saucepan three-fourths full of water to a boil. Add the spaghetti and cook until al dente, 7–9 minutes, or according to package directions. Drain the pasta and rinse in cold running water. Drain again thoroughly and set aside.

In a large bowl, whisk together the soy sauce, vinegar, sesame oil, peanut butter, ginger, garlic, and red pepper flakes. Using your fingers, shred the chicken breasts with the grain into strips about ½ inch (12 mm) thick and about 2 inches (5 cm) long. Add the chicken, pasta, cucumber, carrot, green onions, and cilantro, if using, to the dressing. Toss to combine. Serve at room temperature or chilled.

2 cups (16 fl oz/500 ml) fat-free, no-salt-added chicken broth

1 lb (500 g) skinless, boneless chicken breasts

8 oz (500 g) whole-wheat (wholemeal) or 50-percent whole-wheat spaghetti or other dried pasta

3 tablespoons low-sodium soy sauce

2 tablespoons rice vinegar or white wine vinegar

1 tablespoon dark sesame oil

2 tablespoons creamy natural unsalted peanut butter, stirred well before measuring

1 tablespoon peeled and minced fresh ginger

2 cloves garlic, minced

¼ teaspoon red pepper flakes

1 English (hothouse) cucumber, peeled, cut in half lengthwise, and sliced

1 carrot, peeled and finely shredded

¼ cup (¾ oz/20 g) sliced green (spring) onions

¼ cup (½ oz/15 g) chopped fresh cilantro (fresh coriander) (optional)

NUTRIENT ANALYSIS FOR ONE SERVING

Calories from Fat 20%	**Calories from Carbs** 45%	**Total Fat** 7 g
Protein 25 g	**Carbohydrates** 32 g	**Saturated Fat** 1 g
Sodium 280 mg	**Fiber** 6 g	**Monounsaturated Fat** 3 g
Cholesterol 44 mg	**Sugars** 3 g	**Polyunsaturated Fat** 2 g

PENNE WITH BROCCOLI & GARLIC

SERVES 4

6 oz (185 g) whole-wheat (wholemeal) or 50-percent whole-wheat penne

2 teaspoons olive oil

3 cloves garlic, thinly sliced

1 yellow onion, halved lengthwise and thinly sliced crosswise

¾ cup (6 fl oz/180 ml) fat-free, no-salt-added vegetable or chicken broth

6 cups (12 oz/375 g) broccoli florets

¼ teaspoon red pepper flakes

½ cup (2 oz/60 g) finely shredded Parmesan cheese

If you enjoy the tanginess of bitter greens, try this recipe using leafy broccoli rabe instead of broccoli. Keep in mind that you will need to increase the cooking time to about 10 minutes for broccoli rabe.

Bring a saucepan three-fourths full of water to a boil. Add the penne and cook until al dente, 7–9 minutes, or according to package directions. Drain thoroughly and set aside.

While the pasta is cooking, in a large frying pan, heat the olive oil over medium heat. Add the garlic and cook until the edges begin to brown, about 1 minute. Then add the onion and cook, stirring often, until softened, 4–5 minutes. Add the broth, broccoli, and red pepper flakes. Cover and cook, stirring often, until the broccoli is tender-crisp, about 3 minutes. Add the pasta and stir to mix well.

Divide the pasta mixture among individual bowls. Sprinkle each serving with the Parmesan. Serve immediately.

NUTRIENT ANALYSIS FOR ONE SERVING

Calories from Fat 21%	**Calories from Carbs** 57%	**Total Fat** 8 g
Protein 18 g	**Carbohydrates** 47 g	**Saturated Fat** 3 g
Sodium 301 mg	**Fiber** 8 g	**Monounsaturated Fat** 3 g
Cholesterol 12 mg	**Sugars** 4 g	**Polyunsaturated Fat** 1 g

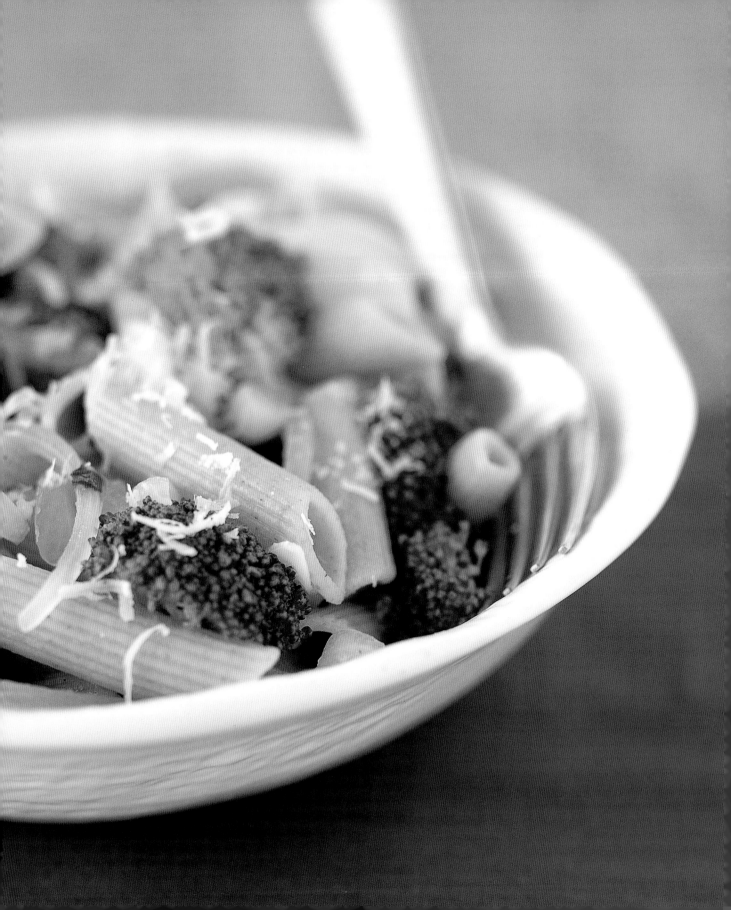

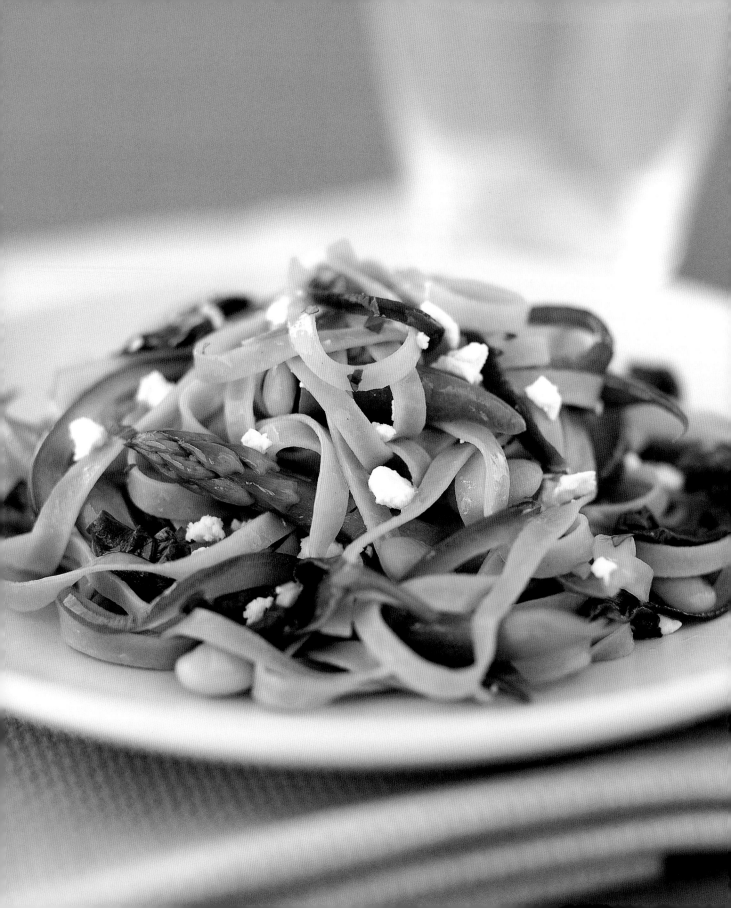

FETTUCCINE WITH SPRING VEGETABLES

CALORIES 353

DIABETIC EXCHANGES

| 3 starch | 0 fruit | 0 milk |
| 1½ vegetable | 2 protein | 2 fat |

SERVES 4

When choosing asparagus, select spears with tightly formed tips and no sign of wilting. Size doesn't matter—large spears are just as tender as thin ones. If you can find ricotta salata cheese, it makes a sharp, tangy substitute for the feta.

Bring a saucepan three-fourths full of water to a boil. Add the pasta and cook for 3 minutes. Stir in the green beans and lima beans and cook for 3 minutes longer. Add the asparagus and cook for 2 minutes longer. Drain thoroughly and set aside.

While the pasta and vegetables are cooking, heat the olive oil in a large frying pan over medium heat. Add the onion and sauté until tender, about 5 minutes. Add the garlic and cook for 1 minute. Stir in the spinach and cook, stirring constantly, until the spinach is wilted, about 1 minute longer. Stir in the pasta and vegetables, and the parsley, if using.

Divide the pasta mixture evenly among individual shallow bowls. Sprinkle with the feta and serve.

8 oz (500 g) whole-wheat (wholemeal) or 50-percent whole-wheat fettuccine, spaghetti, or linguine

½ lb (500 g) green beans, stems trimmed, cut into ½-inch (12-mm) pieces

½ cup (3 oz/90 g) frozen baby lima beans

½ lb (500 g) asparagus spears, tough ends snapped off, cut into 1½-inch (4-cm) pieces

2 tablespoons olive oil

1 red onion, halved lengthwise and thinly sliced crosswise

1 clove garlic, minced

2 cups (4 oz/125 g) chopped fresh spinach or baby spinach leaves

2 tablespoons chopped fresh parsley (optional)

½ cup (2½ oz/75 g) crumbled feta cheese

NUTRIENT ANALYSIS FOR ONE SERVING

Calories from Fat 25%	**Calories from Carbs** 60%	**Total Fat** 10 g
Protein 14 g	**Carbohydrates** 55 g	**Saturated Fat** 3 g
Sodium 190 mg	**Fiber** 12 g	**Monounsaturated Fat** 6 g
Cholesterol 8 mg	**Sugars** 5 g	**Polyunsaturated Fat** 1 g

RATATOUILLE PASTA

SERVES 4

- 8 oz (185 g) whole-wheat (wholemeal) or 50-percent whole-wheat rigatoni or other dried pasta
- 2 tablespoons olive oil
- 1 yellow onion, halved lengthwise and thinly sliced crosswise
- 2 cloves garlic, minced
- 1 eggplant, about 1 lb (500 g), peeled and cut into ½-inch (12-mm) cubes
- 1 red bell pepper (capsicum), chopped
- 1 yellow bell pepper (capsicum), chopped
- 2 tomatoes, chopped
- 1 teaspoon balsamic vinegar
- ½ teaspoon dried basil
- ½ teaspoon dried oregano
- ¼ teaspoon freshly ground pepper
- ¼ cup (1 oz/30 g) finely shredded Parmesan cheese

Ratatouille, a popular French dish that originated in the region of Provence, is a delightful mix of vegetables and herbs. It's low in calories, heart-healthy, and can be served as a main course with pasta, as here, or on its own as a side dish.

Bring a saucepan three-fourths full of water to a boil. Add the rigatoni and cook until al dente, 10–12 minutes, or according to package directions. Drain thoroughly. Set aside.

While the pasta is cooking, in a large, nonstick frying pan, heat the olive oil over medium heat. Add the onion and sauté until tender, about 5 minutes. Add the garlic and cook for 1 minute. Add the eggplant and cook, stirring often, until softened, about 8 minutes. Stir in the bell peppers and tomatoes and cook, stirring often, until the vegetables are almost tender, about 5 minutes longer. Stir in the vinegar, basil, oregano, and pepper and cook until all the vegetables are tender, about 3 minutes longer.

To serve, divide the pasta among individual bowls. Top with the vegetable mixture. Sprinkle each serving with the Parmesan and serve immediately.

NUTRIENT ANALYSIS FOR ONE SERVING

Calories from Fat 28%	**Calories from Carbs** 58%	**Total Fat** 7 g
Protein 8 g	**Carbohydrates** 31 g	**Saturated Fat** 2 g
Sodium 80 mg	Fiber 4 g	**Monounsaturated Fat** 4 g
Cholesterol 4 mg	Sugars 5 g	**Polyunsaturated Fat** 1 g

PORTOBELLOS STUFFED WITH VEGETABLES

SERVES 4

DIABETIC EXCHANGES

1 starch	0 fruit	0 milk
3 vegetable	1 protein	½ fat

No one will miss the meat in this meal of mushrooms, fresh vegetables, and full-flavored Gruyère cheese. Kitchen shears make quick work of slicing the sun-dried tomatoes. A rainbow of peppers and tomatoes, this dish looks as good as it tastes.

Place the bulgur, sun-dried tomatoes, and pepper in a large, heatproof bowl. In a saucepan over high heat, bring 1 cup (8 fl oz/250 ml) of the broth to a boil and pour over the bulgur mixture. Cover the bowl and let stand until the bulgur is tender and the broth is completely absorbed, about 25 minutes.

While the bulgur mixture is soaking, prepare the mushrooms. Using a spoon, gently scrape away and discard the dark gills on the underside of each mushroom. Heat 1 teaspoon of the olive oil in a large, nonstick frying pan over medium-high heat. Add the mushrooms, cover, and cook, turning often, until they are cooked through and tender when pierced with a knife, about 5 minutes. Place the mushrooms, cap side down, in a shallow roasting pan or rimmed baking sheet.

Preheat the broiler (grill). Add 1 teaspoon olive oil to the frying pan. Add the onion and bell peppers and sauté until tender, about 8 minutes. Stir in the garlic and cook for 1 minute. Add the vegetables to the bowl with the bulgur. Add ¼ cup (2 fl oz/60 ml) broth and the parsley and stir to mix well.

Spoon 1 cup (5 oz/155 g) of the bulgur and vegetable mixture into each of the mushroom caps. Sprinkle with the cheese. Place the pan under the broiler and broil (grill) until the cheese is melted, 1–2 minutes. Serve hot.

½ cup (3 oz/90 g) bulgur

½ cup (4 oz/125 g) sun-dried tomato halves, thinly sliced

¼ teaspoon freshly ground pepper

1¼ cups (10 fl oz/310 ml) fat-free, no-salt-added vegetable or chicken broth

4 large portobello mushrooms, brushed clean and stemmed

2 teaspoons olive oil

1 yellow onion, halved lengthwise and thinly sliced crosswise

1 yellow bell pepper (capsicum), cut into short, thin strips

1 red bell pepper (capsicum), cut into short, thin strips

2 cloves garlic, minced

2 tablespoons chopped fresh parsley

¼ cup (1 oz/30 g) shredded Gruyère cheese

NUTRIENT ANALYSIS FOR ONE SERVING

Calories from Fat 23%	**Calories from Carbs** 57%	**Total Fat** 5 g
Protein 10 g	**Carbohydrates** 30 g	**Saturated Fat** 2 g
Sodium 219 mg	**Fiber** 7 g	**Monounsaturated Fat** 3 g
Cholesterol 8 mg	**Sugars** 8 g	**Polyunsaturated Fat** <1 g

VEGETABLE & GOAT CHEESE STRATA

SERVES 6

3 tablespoons goat cheese

1½ cups (12 fl oz/375 ml) 1-percent milk

1 whole egg plus 6 egg whites

½ teaspoon dried oregano

¼ teaspoon freshly ground pepper

7 oz (220 g) sturdy whole-grain bread, cut into ¾-inch (2-cm) cubes (about 5 cups)

1 teaspoon olive oil

1 yellow onion, halved lengthwise and thinly sliced crosswise

1 clove garlic, minced

2 zucchini (courgettes), cut in half lengthwise and thinly sliced

4 cups (8 oz/250 g) chopped fresh spinach or baby spinach leaves

Use day-old bread for making this dish; the bread cubes will be easier to cut and they'll retain their shape better as the casserole bakes. Serve the strata for brunch along with Apple, Raisin & Almond Salad (page 43).

Preheat the oven to 375°F (190°C). Lightly coat an 11-by-7-inch (28-by18-cm) baking dish with olive oil cooking spray.

In a food processor or blender, combine the goat cheese and milk and process until smooth. Transfer to a bowl and stir in the whole egg, egg whites, oregano, and pepper. Add the bread cubes, stir to combine, and let stand while cooking the vegetables.

In a frying pan, heat the olive oil over medium-high heat. Add the onion and sauté until softened, about 5 minutes. Add the garlic and zucchini and cook until the zucchini is tender-crisp, about 5 minutes longer. Stir in the spinach and cook, stirring often, until the spinach is wilted, about 2 minutes longer.

Place half of the bread mixture in the prepared dish. Top with the vegetable mixture, spreading evenly. Cover the vegetable layer with the remaining bread mixture and bake until the top of the strata is lightly browned, about 25 minutes. Let stand for 5 minutes before serving.

NUTRIENT ANALYSIS FOR ONE SERVING

Calories from Fat 25%	**Calories from Carbs** 47%	**Total Fat** 5 g
Protein 12 g	**Carbohydrates** 21 g	**Saturated Fat** 2 g
Sodium 270 mg	**Fiber** 3 g	**Monounsaturated Fat** 2 g
Cholesterol 42 mg	**Sugars** 8 g	**Polyunsaturated Fat** 1 g

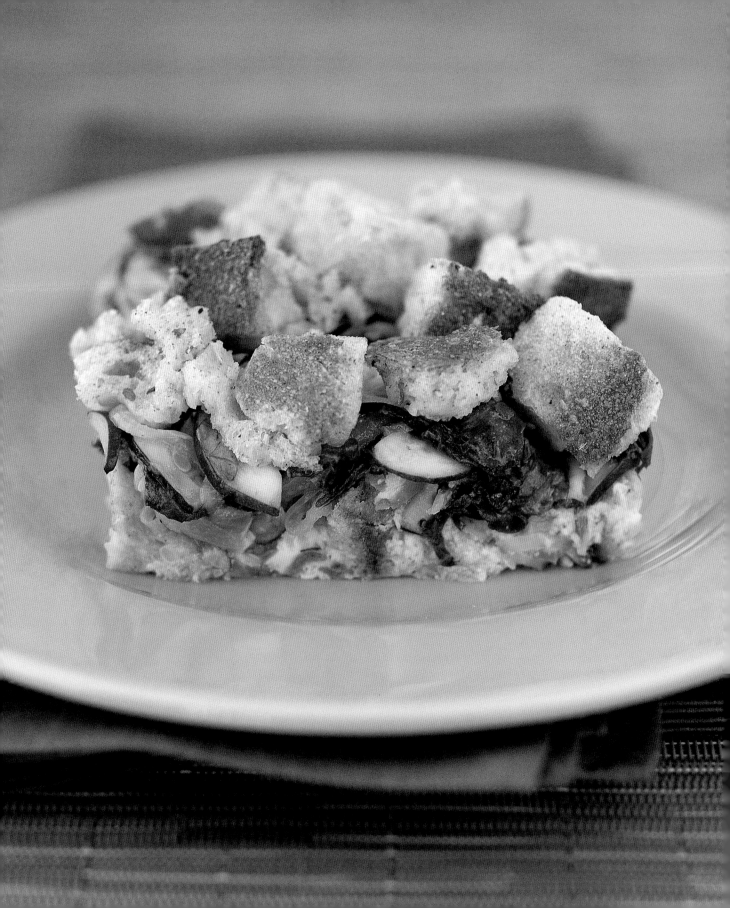

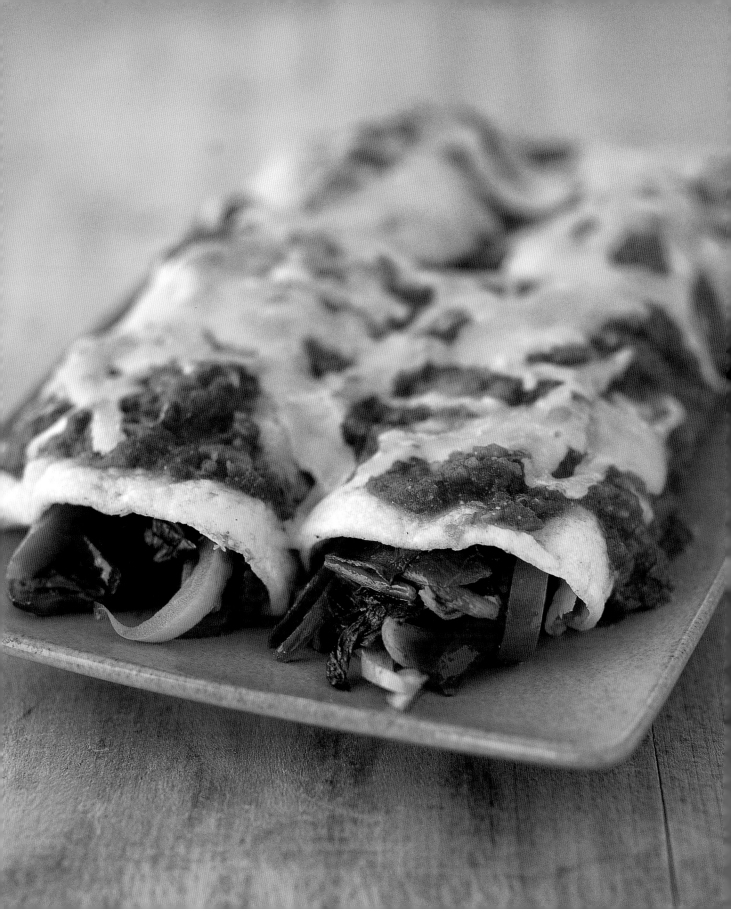

VEGETABLE ENCHILADAS

SERVES 4   Kid-friendly recipe

Filled with vegetables, enchiladas can be a deliciously healthful dinner. These are mild enough for kids, yet flavorful enough for adults. Like all greens, chard is rich in the antioxidant vitamins A and C. If you can't find chard, kale is a good substitute.

Preheat the oven to 375°F (190°C). Coat a 13-by-9-inch (33-by-23-cm) baking dish with 1 teaspoon of the olive oil. Remove the tough stems and ribs of the chard and discard. Coarsely chop the chard greens and set aside. In a large, nonstick frying pan, heat the remaining 1 teaspoon olive oil over medium-high heat. Add the bell peppers and onion and sauté until the vegetables are tender, about 10 minutes. Stir in the garlic and chili powder and cook for 1 minute. Stir in the chard and cook, stirring constantly, until the chard wilts, about 1 minute longer. Remove from the heat and set aside.

In another frying pan, warm the broth over medium heat. Using tongs, carefully dip a tortilla in the broth. Remove immediately and place flat on a work surface. Spoon about ½ cup (3½ oz/105 g) of the vegetable mixture down the center of the tortilla. Roll up and place, seam side down, in the prepared dish. Repeat with the remaining 7 tortillas and filling.

Combine the tomatoes, cilantro, and cumin in a food processor and pulse until finely chopped. Spoon the mixture over the enchiladas. Cover the dish with aluminum foil and bake for 20 minutes. Uncover, sprinkle with the cheese, and bake, uncovered, until the cheese is melted, about 5 minutes longer. Let stand for 5 minutes before serving.

2 teaspoons olive oil

½ lb (250 g) Swiss chard

1 red bell pepper (capsicum), cut into short, thin strips

1 yellow bell pepper (capsicum), cut into short, thin strips

1 yellow onion, halved lengthwise and thinly sliced crosswise

1 clove garlic, minced

2 tablespoons chili powder

1 cup (8 fl oz/250 ml) fat-free, no-salt-added vegetable or chicken broth

Eight 6-inch (15-cm) corn tortillas

One 14-oz (440-g) can no-salt-added diced tomatoes

½ cup (½ oz/15 g) whole fresh cilantro (fresh coriander) leaves or 1 teaspoon ground coriander

½ teaspoon ground cumin

½ cup (2 oz/60 g) shredded reduced-fat Colby cheese

NUTRIENT ANALYSIS FOR ONE SERVING

Calories from Fat 21%	**Calories from Carbs** 63%	**Total Fat** 6 g
Protein 10 g	**Carbohydrates** 37 g	**Saturated Fat** 1 g
Sodium 248 mg	**Fiber** 8 g	**Monounsaturated Fat** 3 g
Cholesterol 3 mg	**Sugars** 7 g	**Polyunsaturated Fat** 1 g

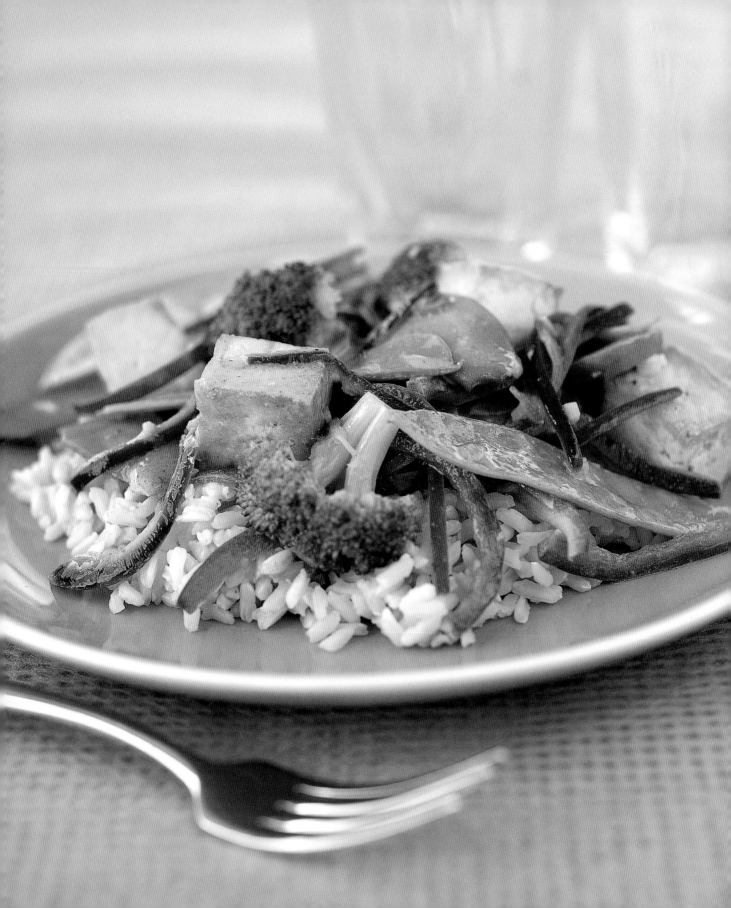

CURRIED TOFU & VEGETABLE STIR-FRY

CALORIES 257

SERVES 4

Curry paste, an aromatic and flavorful blend of chiles and Thai spices, is worth seeking out. Look for jars of red or green curry paste in the Asian section of well-stocked supermarkets. If you can't find the paste, curry powder is an acceptable substitute.

Gently press the tofu cubes between layers of paper towels to remove excess moisture. Set aside. In a bowl, combine the coconut milk, curry paste, and lime juice and stir to mix well. Set aside.

In a large, nonstick frying pan, heat 1 teaspoon of the oil over medium-high heat. Add the tofu and cook, stirring often, until lightly browned, 5–6 minutes. Transfer to a plate. Add the remaining 1 teaspoon oil to the same pan. Add the ginger and garlic and toss and stir constantly until fragrant, about 30 seconds. Add the carrot and onion and toss and stir constantly until slightly softened, about 2 minutes. Add the bell pepper, broccoli, and snow peas and toss and stir constantly until slightly softened, about 3 minutes. Add the coconut-milk mixture and toss and stir constantly until the mixture comes to a boil, about 30 seconds. Serve immediately, with the rice.

8 oz (250 g) firm reduced-fat tofu, cut into ¾-inch (2-cm) cubes

⅔ cup (5 fl oz/160 ml) reduced-fat coconut milk

2 teaspoons green curry paste, 1 teaspoon red curry paste, or 2 teaspoons curry powder

1 tablespoon fresh lime juice

2 teaspoons canola oil

1 tablespoon peeled and minced fresh ginger

2 cloves garlic, minced

1 carrot, peeled and sliced

1 red onion, halved lengthwise and thinly sliced crosswise

1 red bell pepper (capsicum), cut into short, thin strips

2 cups (4 oz/125 g) broccoli florets

1 cup (5 oz/155 g) fresh snow peas (mangetouts)

2 cups (10 oz/315 g) cooked brown rice

NUTRIENT ANALYSIS FOR ONE SERVING

Calories from Fat 27%	**Calories from Carbs** 56%	**Total Fat** 8 g
Protein 12 g	**Carbohydrates** 37 g	**Saturated Fat** 2 g
Sodium 88 mg	**Fiber** 6 g	**Monounsaturated Fat** 2 g
Cholesterol 0 mg	**Sugars** 4 g	**Polyunsaturated Fat** 1 g

ARTICHOKE & SPINACH FRITTATA

DIABETIC EXCHANGES

0 starch	0 fruit	0 milk
1½ vegetable	2 protein	½ fat

SERVES 4

1 whole egg plus 9 egg whites

1 teaspoon olive oil

1 small yellow onion, diced

1 clove garlic, minced

One 9-oz (280-g) package frozen artichoke hearts, thawed and quartered

3 cups (6 oz/185 g) chopped fresh spinach or baby spinach leaves

¼ teaspoon freshly ground pepper

2 tablespoons grated Parmesan cheese

When you make a frittata using mostly cholesterol-free egg whites and lots of vegetables, it's a nutrient-dense, low-fat brunch, lunch, or light supper. Using frozen artichokes takes the work out of preparing this otherwise labor-intensive vegetable.

Preheat the broiler (grill).

In a bowl, whisk together the whole egg and the egg whites. Set aside.

In a large nonstick frying pan with an ovenproof handle, heat the olive oil over medium heat. Add the onion and sauté until tender, about 5 minutes. Add the garlic and cook for 1 minute. Stir in the artichokes and spinach and cook, stirring constantly, until the artichokes are heated through and the spinach is wilted, about 2 minutes. Stir in the pepper. Pour the egg mixture into the pan with the vegetables and cook for 30 seconds. Use a spatula to push the edges of the egg towards the center, allowing the uncooked egg to seep to the bottom of the pan, and continue cooking until the bottom of the frittata is set, about 2 minutes.

Sprinkle the frittata with the Parmesan. Carefully place the pan under the broiler and broil (grill) until the frittata is lightly browned and completely set, about 2 minutes. Gently slide onto a warmed serving platter and cut into wedges. Serve immediately.

NUTRIENT ANALYSIS FOR ONE SERVING

Calories from Fat 26%	**Calories from Carbs** 31%	**Total Fat** 4 g
Protein 14 g	**Carbohydrates** 10 g	**Saturated Fat** 1 g
Sodium 233 mg	**Fiber** 4 g	**Monounsaturated Fat** 2 g
Cholesterol 55 mg	**Sugars** 2 g	**Polyunsaturated Fat** 0 g

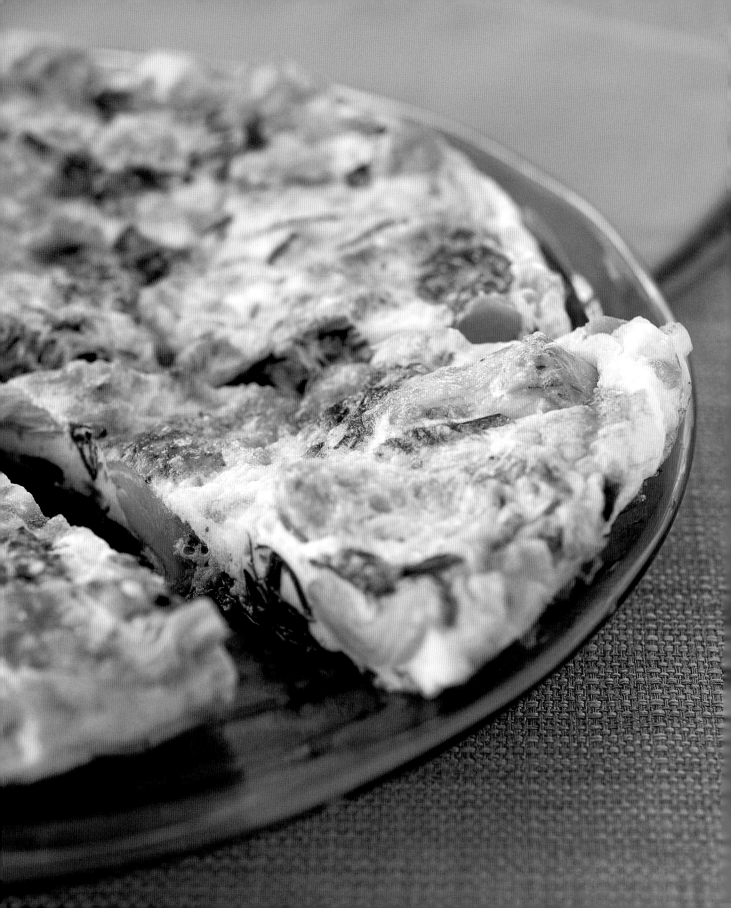

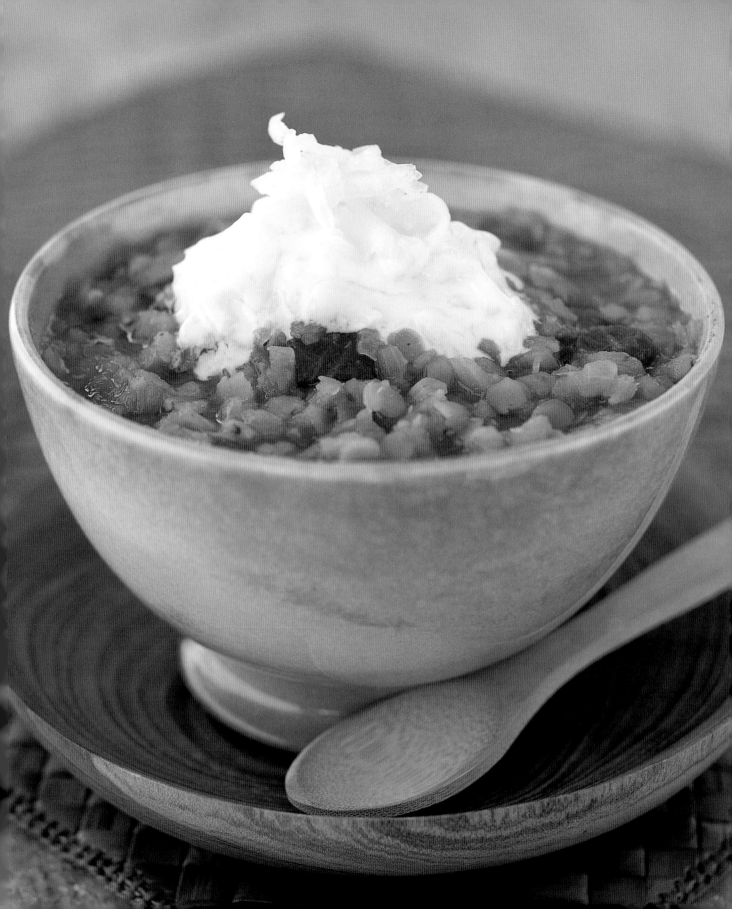

SPICED LENTILS

SERVES 4

If you wish, use 2 tablespoons of curry powder instead of the mixture of ground spices called for to season this dish. Brown lentils are a widely available alternative to red lentils— just simmer them for about 5 minutes longer.

In a large saucepan, heat the olive oil over medium heat. Add the onion and sauté until tender, about 5 minutes. Stir in the garlic, ginger, cumin, coriander, turmeric, and cayenne, if using, and cook for 1 minute. Stir in the broth, tomatoes, and lentils. Cover and bring to a boil over high heat. Reduce the heat to medium-low and simmer, covered, until the lentils are tender, 10–15 minutes.

While the lentils are cooking, combine the yogurt, cucumber, and lime juice in a small bowl and stir to mix well.

To serve, ladle the lentils into individual bowls and top each serving with about 2 tablespoons of the cucumber-yogurt sauce.

2 tablespoons olive oil

1 yellow onion, diced

1 clove garlic, minced

2 teaspoons ground ginger

2 teaspoons ground cumin

1 teaspoon ground coriander

1 teaspoon ground turmeric

⅛ teaspoon cayenne pepper (optional)

3 cups (24 fl oz/750 ml) fat-free, no-salt-added vegetable or chicken broth

One 14-oz (440-g) can no-salt-added diced tomatoes

1 cup (7 oz/220 g) red lentils, rinsed

¼ cup (2 oz/60 g) plain low-fat yogurt

¼ cup (1½ oz/15 g) peeled, seeded, and shredded cucumber

2 teaspoons fresh lime juice

NUTRIENT ANALYSIS FOR ONE SERVING

Calories from Fat 24%	**Calories from Carbs** 51%	**Total Fat** 8 g
Protein 19 g	**Carbohydrates** 38 g	**Saturated Fat** 1 g
Sodium 155 mg	**Fiber** 17 g	**Monounsaturated Fat** 6 g
Cholesterol 1 mg	**Sugars** 8 g	**Polyunsaturated Fat** 1 g

WHITE BEAN & BACON STEW

SERVES 6

2 strips reduced-sodium bacon

1 yellow onion, chopped

2 celery stalks, chopped

2 carrots, peeled and chopped

2 cloves garlic, minced

4 cups (32 fl oz/1 l) fat-free, no-salt-added chicken broth

Three 15-oz (470-g) cans no-salt-added cannellini beans, rinsed and drained

3 tomatoes, chopped

2 teaspoons minced fresh rosemary or 2 teaspoons crumbled dried rosemary

½ teaspoon freshly ground pepper

A little bit of bacon goes a long way in flavoring this robust stew. Serve it on a chilly night with crusty whole-grain bread and a crisp green salad. If fresh tomatoes are out of season, substitute a 14-oz (440-g) can of no-salt-added diced tomatoes.

In a large pot, cook the bacon over medium heat until crisp, 4–5 minutes. Transfer to a paper towel to drain. Pour off and discard all but 1 teaspoon of the drippings from the pot.

Add the onion, celery, and carrots to the pot and cook, stirring occasionally, until softened, about 5 minutes. Stir in the garlic and cook for 1 minute.

Add the broth and beans and bring to a boil over high heat. Reduce the heat to low and simmer, covered, stirring occasionally, until the vegetables are tender, about 8 minutes. Chop the bacon and stir into the soup along with the tomatoes, rosemary, and pepper. Simmer, uncovered, until the tomatoes are heated through, about 3 minutes longer. Ladle into individual bowls and serve immediately.

NUTRIENT ANALYSIS FOR ONE SERVING

Calories from Fat 14%	**Calories from Carbs** 60%	**Total Fat** 4 g
Protein 16 g	**Carbohydrates** 37 g	**Saturated Fat** 1 g
Sodium 213 mg	**Fiber** 11 g	**Monounsaturated Fat** 1 g
Cholesterol 4 mg	**Sugars** 6 g	**Polyunsaturated Fat** 0 g

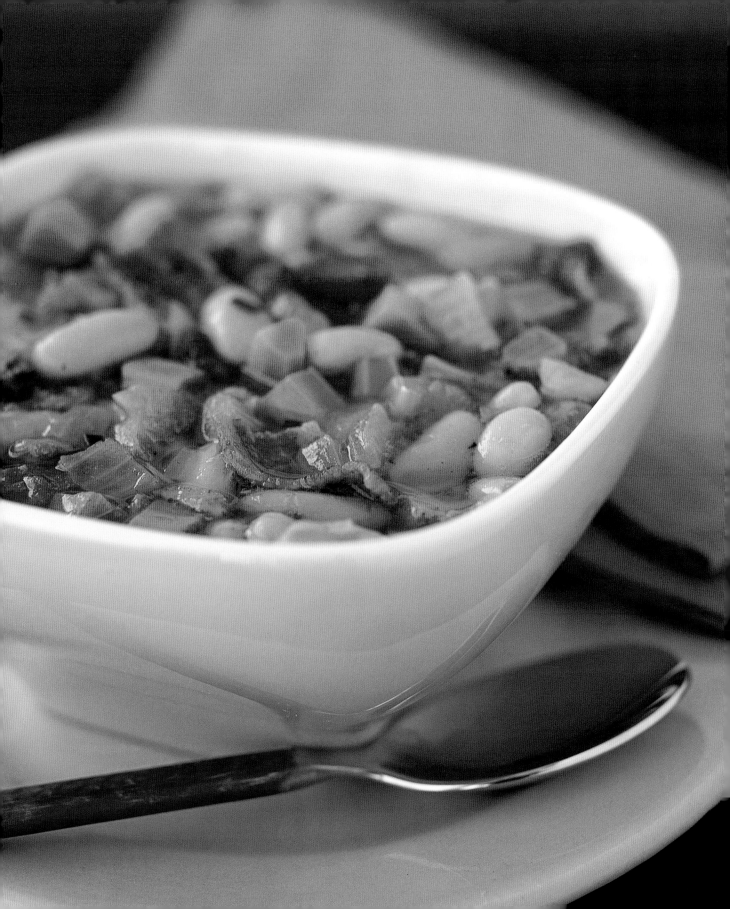

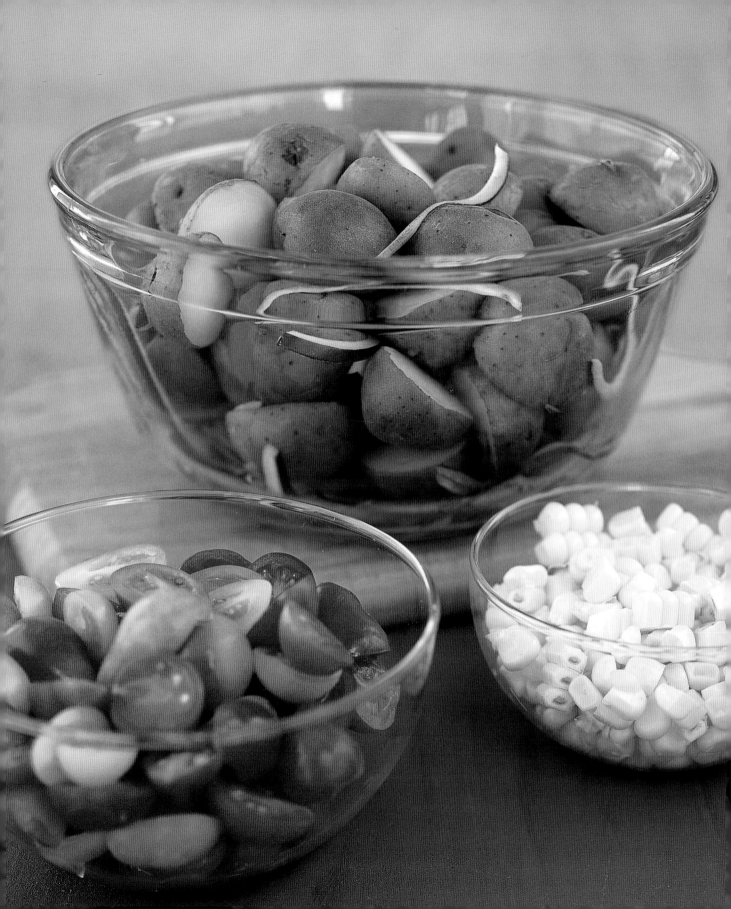

SIDE DISHES

New Potato Salad with Summer Vegetables, 112

SWEET POTATO OVEN FRIES

SERVES 4

Kid-friendly recipe

2 large sweet potatoes, about 1½ lb (750 g) total weight

1 tablespoon olive oil

Let your imagination go wild when seasoning these "fries." Try nutmeg, ground cinnamon or ginger, or a spice blend like Chinese five-spice powder. Serve them with Cheddar Turkey Burgers (page 65) or roasted pork tenderloin.

Preheat the oven to 400°F (200°C).

Peel the sweet potatoes and cut each one in half crosswise. Cut each half lengthwise into two pieces, then slice each of these pieces into four wedges about 2½ inches (6 cm) long. Place the wedges in a shallow roasting pan or rimmed baking sheet and drizzle with the olive oil. Toss to coat and arrange the wedges in a single layer.

Bake, turning once, until tender and lightly browned, about 35 minutes. Serve immediately.

NUTRIENT ANALYSIS FOR ONE SERVING

Calories from Fat 26%	Calories from Carbs 68%	Total Fat 4 g
Protein 2 g	Carbohydrates 21 g	Saturated Fat 1 g
Sodium 37 mg	Fiber 3 g	Monounsaturated Fat 3 g
Cholesterol 0 mg	Sugars 9 g	Polyunsaturated Fat 0 g

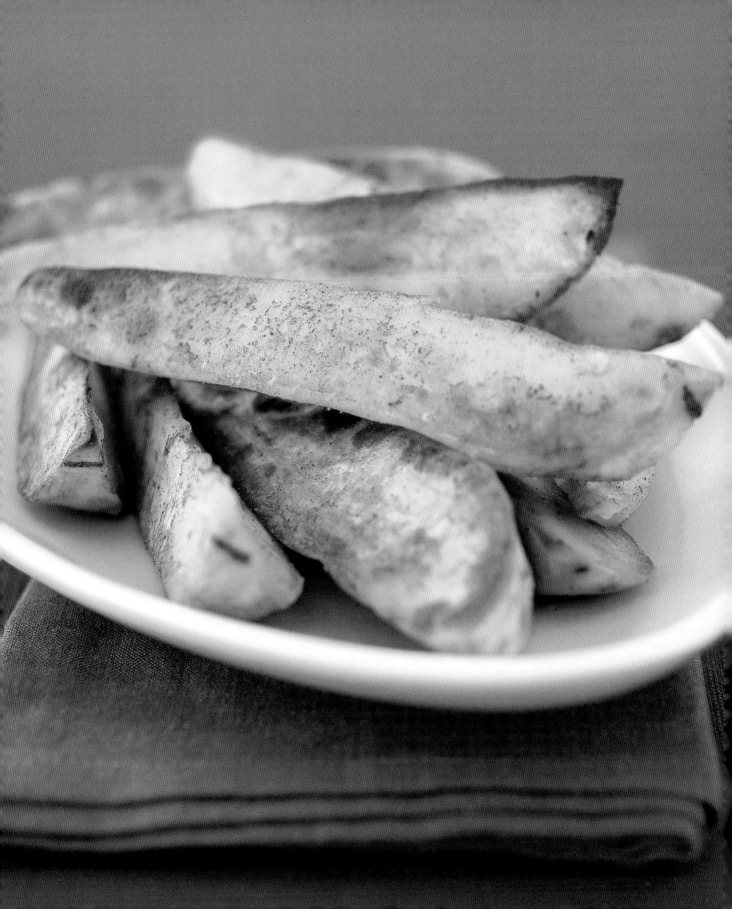

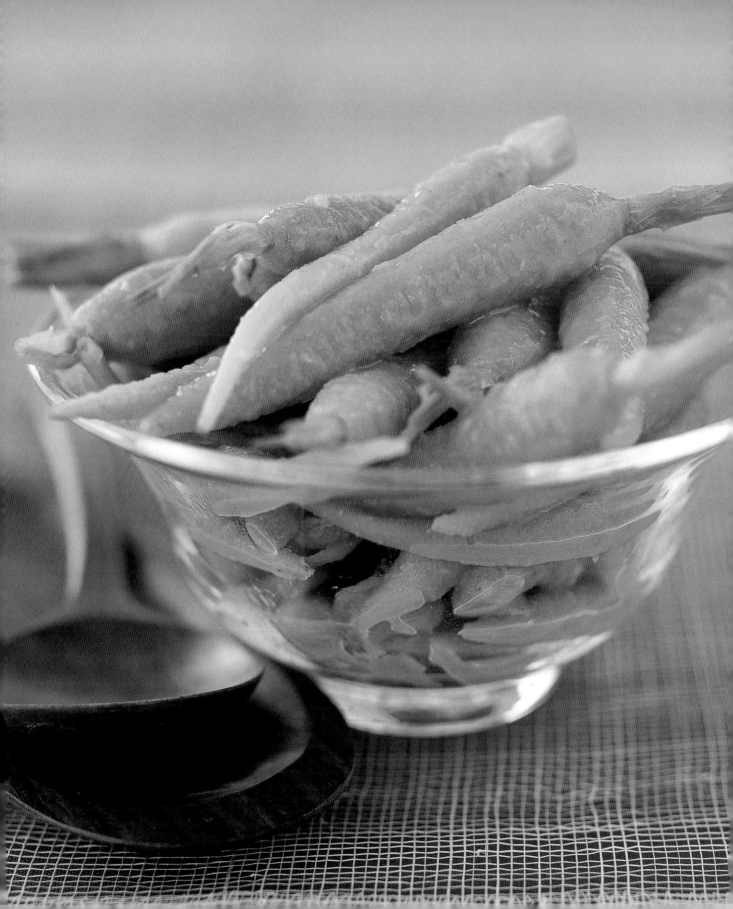

BABY CARROTS WITH ORANGE GLAZE

SERVES 4   Kid-friendly recipe

Look for fresh, tender baby carrots with the green tops still attached. (Those sold in plastic bags are large, less-tender carrots that have been cut into pieces.) These beta carotene–boosting carrots make a kid-pleasing side dish to roast chicken.

In a saucepan, combine the carrots and orange juice. Cover and bring to a boil over high heat. Reduce the heat to medium-low and simmer until the carrots are almost tender, about 6 minutes. Uncover and cook until the carrots are tender and the orange juice is thickened to a glaze consistency, about 2 minutes.

Remove from the heat and stir in the olive oil and orange zest. Serve immediately.

1 lb (500 g) baby carrots

½ cup (4 fl oz/125 ml) fresh orange juice

1 teaspoon olive oil

1 teaspoon grated orange zest

NUTRIENT ANALYSIS FOR ONE SERVING

Calories from Fat 19%	**Calories from Carbs** 76%	**Total Fat** 1 g
Protein 1 g	**Carbohydrates** 13 g	**Saturated Fat** 0 g
Sodium 89 mg	**Fiber** 2 g	**Monounsaturated Fat** 1 g
Cholesterol 0 mg	**Sugars** 8 g	**Polyunsaturated Fat** 0 g

DIABETIC EXCHANGES

1 starch	0 fruit	0 milk
0 vegetable	½ protein	0 fat

SERVES 6

Kid-friendly recipe

1½ lb (750 g) unpeeled Yukon gold potatoes, scrubbed and cut into 1-inch (2.5-cm) cubes

2 cloves garlic, chopped

2 cups (16 fl oz/500 ml) fat-free, no-salt-added vegetable or chicken broth

¾ cup (6 fl oz/180 ml) 1-percent milk

1 tablespoon minced fresh chives or 1 tablespoon minced green (spring) onions

¼ teaspoon freshly ground pepper

You can make this dish with russet potatoes, but the moist texture and earthy flavor of Yukon gold potatoes make them worth seeking out. You can omit the garlic, if you wish, to please young palates.

In a saucepan, combine the potatoes, garlic, and broth. Cover and bring to a boil over high heat. Reduce the heat to medium-low and simmer until the potatoes are tender, 10–12 minutes.

Drain the potatoes in a colander, then return them to the same saucepan. Add the milk and, using a potato masher or handheld mixer, mash the potatoes until light and fluffy. Stir in the chives and pepper. Serve immediately.

NUTRIENT ANALYSIS FOR ONE SERVING

Calories from Fat 4%	**Calories from Carbs** 81%	**Total Fat** <1 g
Protein 4 g	**Carbohydrates** 20 g	**Saturated Fat** 0 g
Sodium 42 mg	**Fiber** 3 g	**Monounsaturated Fat** 0 g
Cholesterol 2 mg	**Sugars** 3 g	**Polyunsaturated Fat** 0 g

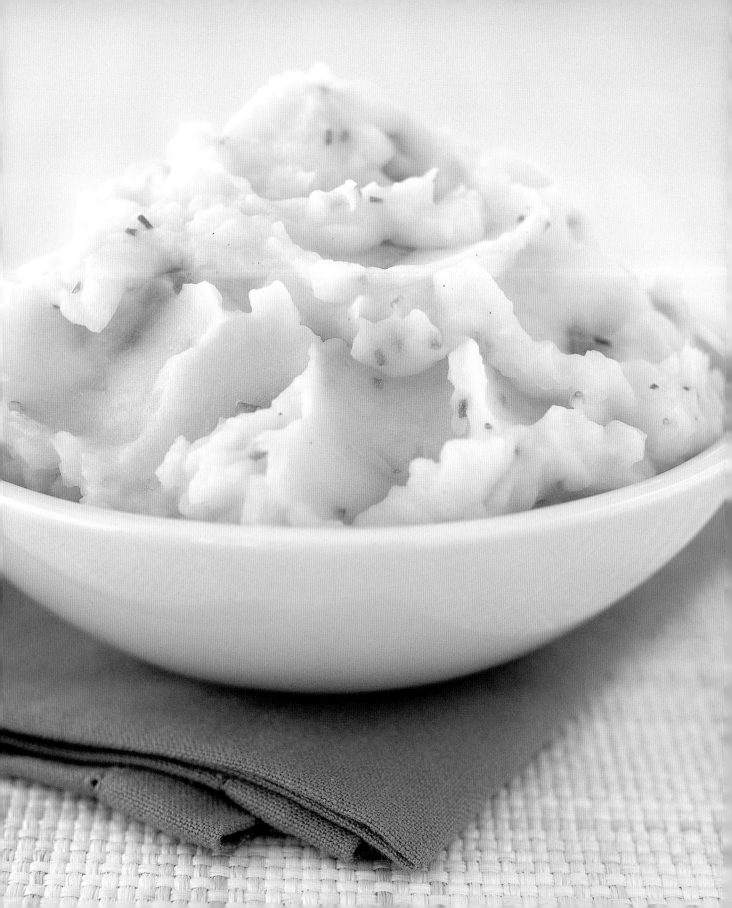

BUTTERNUT SQUASH WITH SAGE

SERVES 4

2 teaspoons olive oil

1 butternut squash, about 2 lb, (1 kg), peeled and cut into 1-inch (2.5-cm) cubes

1 teaspoon chopped fresh sage or 1 teaspoon dried sage leaves

¼ teaspoon freshly ground pepper

To easily prepare the squash, cut it in half crosswise using a strong, sharp, serrated knife. Cut each half in half again lengthwise, remove the seeds, and peel using a vegetable peeler. Use rosemary instead of sage in this dish if you prefer.

In a large, nonstick frying pan, heat the olive oil over medium-high heat. Add the squash, cover, and cook, stirring often, until tender and lightly browned, 10–12 minutes.

Stir in the sage and pepper and serve immediately.

NUTRIENT ANALYSIS FOR ONE SERVING

Calories from Fat 16%	**Calories from Carbs** 77%	**Total Fat** 3 g
Protein 2 g	**Carbohydrates** 28 g	**Saturated Fat** 0 g
Sodium 10 mg	**Fiber** 5 g	**Monounsaturated Fat** 2 g
Cholesterol 0 mg	**Sugars** 5 g	**Polyunsaturated Fat** 0 g

WILD RICE SALAD WITH GRAPES

DIABETIC EXCHANGES

2 starch	½ fruit	0 milk
0 vegetable	1 protein	½ fat

SERVES 6

Recent commercial production in California and the Midwest has brought the price of wild rice down slightly, but it is still a somewhat expensive indulgence. When you are watching your budget, use 1 cup (7 oz/220 g) uncooked brown rice instead of wild rice.

In a saucepan, combine the rice and 2½ cups (20 fl oz/625 ml) water. Cover and bring to a boil over high heat. Reduce the heat to medium-low and simmer until the rice is tender, about 30 minutes. If any water remains in the pan, drain the rice. Set aside.

Meanwhile, put the almonds in a small, dry, nonstick frying pan over medium-low heat and cook, stirring constantly, until lightly toasted, about 2 minutes. Transfer to a plate and set aside.

In a large bowl, combine the orange zest and juice, vinegar, olive oil, and pepper. Whisk to blend. Add the warm rice to the vinaigrette and toss gently to coat. Let cool to room temperature, then stir in the green onions and grapes. Stir in the toasted almonds just before serving. Serve at room temperature or chilled.

1½ cups (9 oz/280 g) wild rice

¼ cup (1 oz/30 g) sliced (flaked) almonds

2 teaspoons grated orange zest

⅓ cup (3 fl oz/80 ml) fresh orange juice

½ teaspoon cider vinegar

2 teaspoons olive oil

¼ teaspoon freshly ground pepper

2 tablespoons thinly sliced green (spring) onions

¾ cup (4½ oz/140 g) red seedless grapes, halved

NUTRIENT ANALYSIS FOR ONE SERVING

Calories from Fat 18%	**Calories from Carbs** 69%	**Total Fat** 4 g
Protein 7 g	**Carbohydrates** 34 g	**Saturated Fat** 0 g
Sodium 4 mg	**Fiber** 3 g	**Monounsaturated Fat** 3 g
Cholesterol 0 mg	**Sugars** 5 g	**Polyunsaturated Fat** 1 g

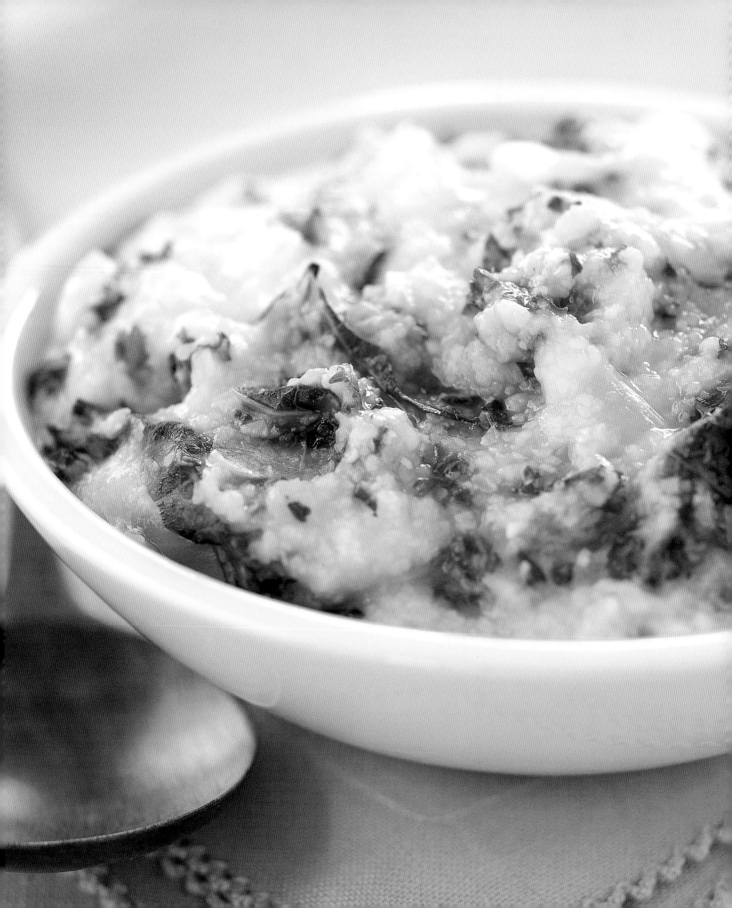

CREAMY POLENTA WITH KALE & PARMESAN

CALORIES 131

DIABETIC EXCHANGES
| 1 starch | 0 fruit | 0 milk |
| 1 vegetable | 1 protein | 0 fat |

SERVES 6

Polenta is foolproof and quick to make when you use the instant variety. This recipe is especially easy, since the greens cook in the same pot with the polenta. Serve with Roasted Pork Loin with Acorn Squash (page 71) or a roast chicken.

Remove the tough stems and ribs of the kale and discard. Coarsely chop the kale greens and set them aside.

In a large saucepan, heat the olive oil over medium heat. Add the onion and sauté until tender, about 5 minutes. Add the garlic and cook for 1 minute. Add the broth, cover, and bring to a boil over medium-high heat. Stir in the kale and cook for 2 minutes. Gradually add the polenta, stirring constantly to avoid lumps. Cook, still stirring constantly, until the broth is absorbed and the polenta is creamy, about 2 minutes. Remove from the heat and stir in the Parmesan and pepper. Serve immediately.

½ lb (500 g) kale or Swiss chard

1 teaspoon olive oil

1 yellow onion, diced

1 clove garlic, minced

3 cups (24 fl oz/750 ml) fat-free, no-salt-added vegetable or chicken broth

¾ cup (5 oz/155 g) instant polenta or fine-grind yellow cornmeal

¼ cup (1 oz/30 g) grated Parmesan cheese

¼ teaspoon freshly ground pepper

NUTRIENT ANALYSIS FOR ONE SERVING

Calories from Fat 13%	Calories from Carbs 67%	Total Fat 2 g
Protein 7 g	Carbohydrates 22 g	Saturated Fat 1 g
Sodium 125 mg	Fiber 3 g	Monounsaturated Fat 1 g
Cholesterol 3 mg	Sugars 1 g	Polyunsaturated Fat 0 g

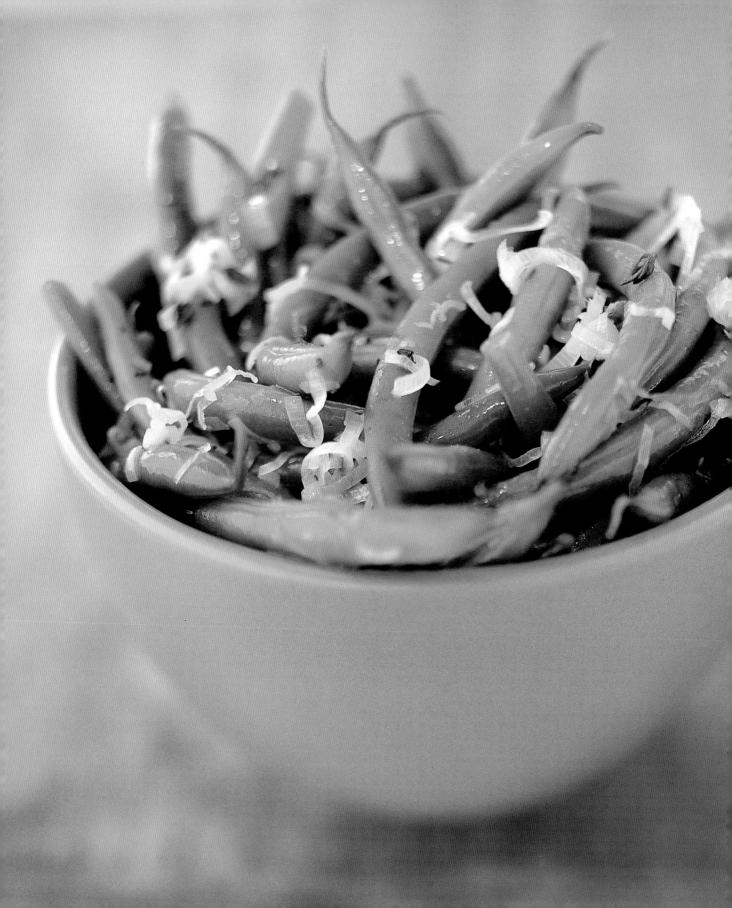

GREEN BEANS WITH LEEKS & THYME

SERVES 4

To make sure you remove all the sandy grit from leeks, cut them in half lengthwise and then rinse them thoroughly under cool water. This dish is a perfect accompaniment to Herb-Crusted Chicken (page 60).

In a large, nonstick frying pan, heat the olive oil over medium heat. Add the leek and sauté until softened and lightly browned, about 7 minutes.

Meanwhile, in a saucepan fitted with a steamer basket, bring 1 inch (2.5 cm) of water to a boil. Add the green beans, cover, and steam until tender, 3–5 minutes, depending on the beans' thickness.

Add the beans, broth, thyme, and pepper to the pan with the leeks. Cook, stirring often, until most of the broth evaporates, about 1 minute. Serve immediately.

1 teaspoon olive oil

1 large leek, about ½ lb (250 g), cut in half lengthwise and thinly sliced

1 lb (500 g) green beans, stems trimmed

¼ cup (2 fl oz/60 ml) fat-free, no-salt-added vegetable or chicken broth

1 tablespoon chopped fresh thyme or 1 teaspoon dried thyme

¼ teaspoon freshly ground pepper

NUTRIENT ANALYSIS FOR ONE SERVING

Calories from Fat 19%	**Calories from Carbs** 66%	**Total Fat** 1 g
Protein 3 g	**Carbohydrates** 11 g	**Saturated Fat** 0 g
Sodium 19 mg	**Fiber** 4 g	**Monounsaturated Fat** 1 g
Cholesterol 0 mg	**Sugars** 2 g	**Polyunsaturated Fat** 0 g

DIABETIC EXCHANGES

1 starch	0 fruit	0 milk
0 vegetable	0 protein	0 fat

SERVES 6

2 teaspoons olive oil

1 lb (500 g) sugar snap peas,
trimmed of stems and strings, or
one 8-oz (250-g) box frozen sugar
snap peas, thawed

1 lb (500 g) English peas, shelled
(about 1 cup/5 oz/155 g), or about
1 cup (5 oz/155 g) frozen shelled
peas, thawed

1 tablespoon chopped fresh mint
or parsley

When peas are at their peak in early spring, this simple dish showcases their garden-fresh flavor. It's almost as good with frozen peas, so you can enjoy it at any time of the year. Serve with Pan-Seared Tuna with Cucumber-Lemon Relish (page 58).

In a large frying pan, heat the olive oil over medium heat. Add the sugar snap peas, cover, and cook, stirring occasionally, until almost tender-crisp, 3–4 minutes. Add the English peas and cook, uncovered, stirring often, until all the peas are tender, 2–3 minutes longer. Stir in the mint and serve immediately.

NUTRIENT ANALYSIS FOR ONE SERVING

Calories from Fat 19%	**Calories from Carbs** 61%	**Total Fat** 2 g
Protein 4 g	**Carbohydrates** 12 g	**Saturated Fat** 0 g
Sodium 80 mg	**Fiber** 4 g	**Monounsaturated Fat** 1 g
Cholesterol 0 mg	**Sugars** 6 g	**Polyunsaturated Fat** 0 g

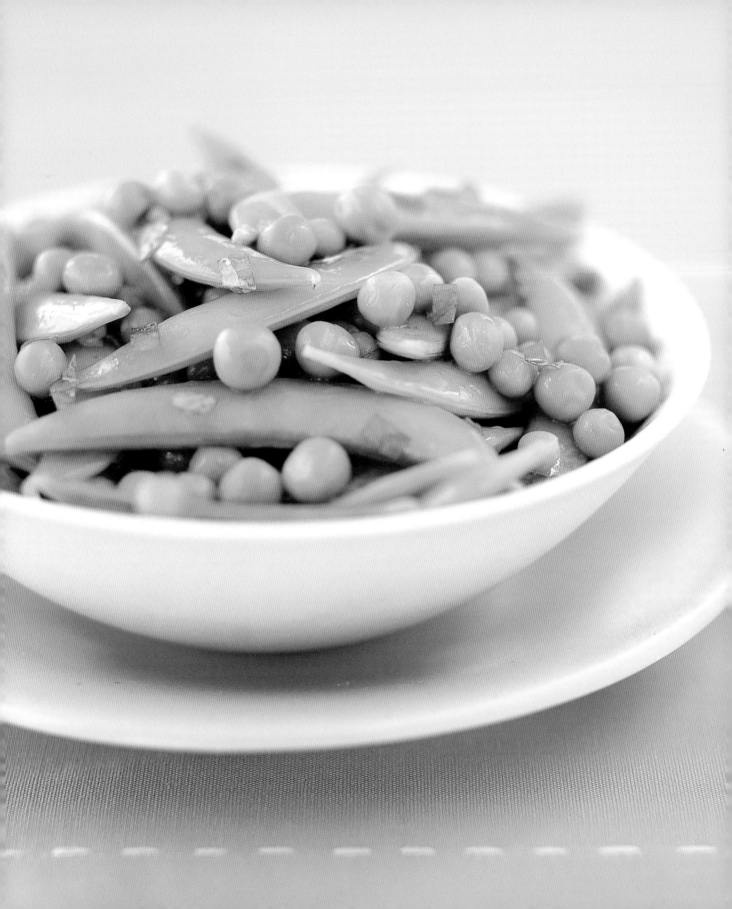

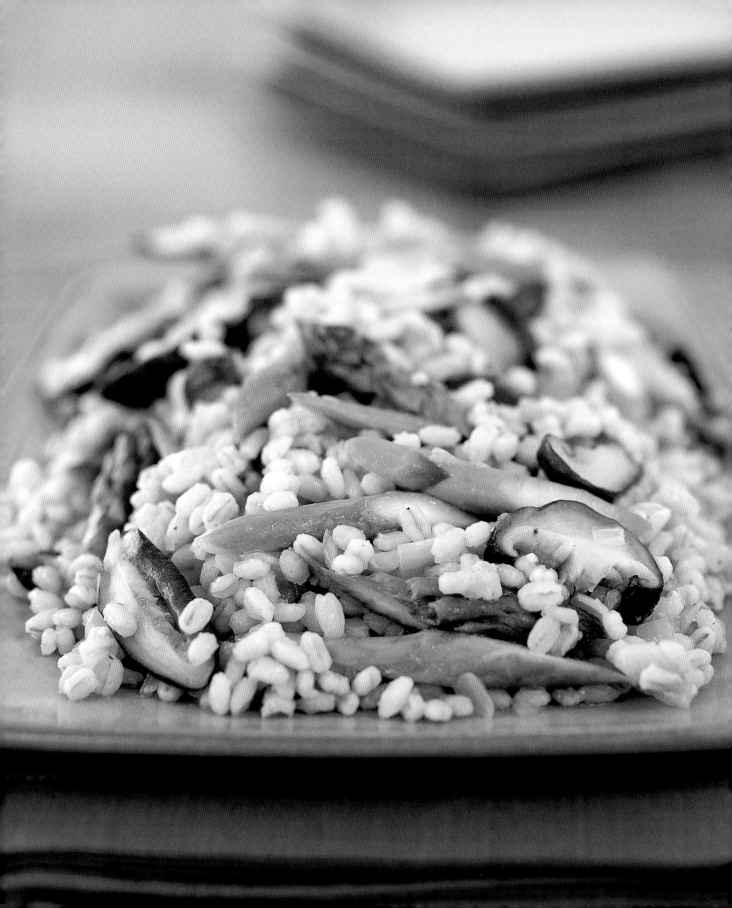

BARLEY, ASPARAGUS & MUSHROOM PILAF

DIABETIC EXCHANGES

1 starch	0 fruit	0 milk
2 vegetable	½ protein	½ fat

SERVES 4

Fresh asparagus and shiitake mushrooms complement the subtle flavor of fiber-rich barley. Use regular button mushrooms if shiitakes are not available. Pair this dish with a crisp green salad for a complete and satisfying vegetarian meal.

In a saucepan, heat 1 teaspoon of the olive oil over medium heat. Add the onion and sauté until it begins to soften, about 3 minutes. Add the garlic and the barley and cook, stirring constantly, for 2 minutes. Stir in the broth. Raise the heat to medium-high, cover, and bring to a boil. Reduce the heat to low and simmer, stirring often during the last 5 minutes of cooking, until the broth is absorbed and the barley is tender, about 25 minutes.

When the barley is almost tender, heat the remaining 1 teaspoon olive oil in a nonstick frying pan over medium heat. Add the asparagus and mushrooms and sauté until tender-crisp, about 4 minutes. Add the vegetables and the pepper to the barley mixture and stir gently to combine. Serve immediately.

2 teaspoons olive oil

½ cup (2 oz/60 g) diced yellow onion

1 clove garlic, minced

½ cup (3½ oz/105 g) pearl barley

2½ cups (20 fl oz/625 ml) fat-free, no-salt-added vegetable or chicken broth

½ lb (250 g) asparagus spears, tough ends snapped off, cut into 1-inch (2.5-cm) pieces

4 oz (125 g) shiitake mushrooms, brushed clean, stemmed, and sliced

¼ teaspoon freshly ground pepper

NUTRIENT ANALYSIS FOR ONE SERVING

Calories from Fat 15%	**Calories from Carbs** 75%	**Total Fat** 3 g
Protein 4 g	**Carbohydrates** 31 g	**Saturated Fat** 0 g
Sodium 211 mg	**Fiber** 6 g	**Monounsaturated Fat** 2 g
Cholesterol 0 mg	**Sugars** 4 g	**Polyunsaturated Fat** 0 g

NEW POTATO SALAD WITH SUMMER VEGETABLES

SERVES 4

1 lb (500 g) small potatoes, about 1-inch (2.5-cm) diameter

2 tablespoons fat-free, no-salt-added vegetable or chicken broth

1 tablespoon white wine vinegar

2 teaspoons olive oil

½ teaspoon freshly ground pepper

½ cup (3 oz/90 g) fresh or thawed frozen corn kernels

1 cup (6 oz/185 g) cherry tomatoes, halved

¼ cup (1 oz/30 g) thinly sliced red onion

2 tablespoons chopped fresh parsley

If small potatoes are not available, use regular red-skinned potatoes: cook them whole and unpeeled, cut them into bite-sized pieces, and proceed with the recipe as directed. Make a double batch of this salad to take to a potluck or picnic.

In a saucepan fitted with a steamer basket, bring 1 inch (2.5 cm) of water to a boil. Add the potatoes, cover, and steam until tender, about 10 minutes. Let cool slightly and cut each potato in half.

While the potatoes are steaming, in a large bowl, whisk together the broth, vinegar, olive oil, and pepper. Place the warm potatoes in the bowl with the vinaigrette, stir once to coat, and let cool to room temperature.

Add the corn, tomatoes, onion, and parsley to the cooled potatoes and toss gently to mix. Serve at room temperature or chilled.

NUTRIENT ANALYSIS FOR ONE SERVING

Calories from Fat 19%	**Calories from Carbs** 72%	**Total Fat** 3 g
Protein 3 g	**Carbohydrates** 25 g	**Saturated Fat** 0 g
Sodium 25 mg	**Fiber** 3 g	**Monounsaturated Fat** 2 g
Cholesterol 0 mg	**Sugars** 3 g	**Polyunsaturated Fat** 0 g

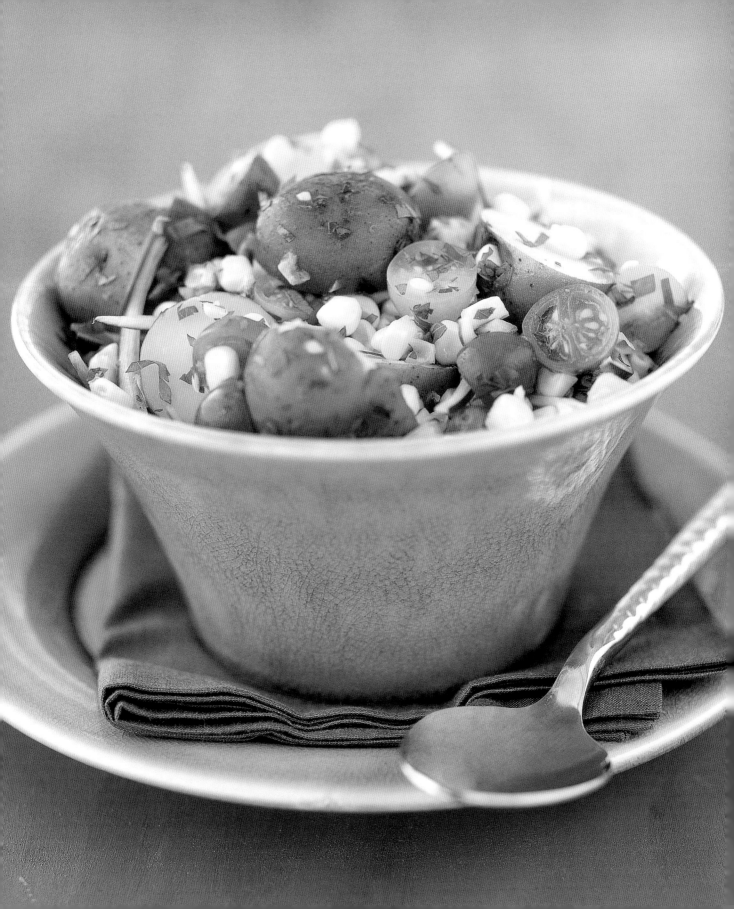

MASHED ROOT VEGETABLES

SERVES 6

2 parsnips, about ¾ lb (12 oz/375 g) total weight, peeled and chopped

1 clove garlic, chopped

3 cups (24 fl oz/750 ml) fat-free, no-salt-added vegetable or chicken broth

2 sweet potatoes, about 1½ lb (24 oz/750 g) total weight, peeled and chopped

2 turnips, about 1 lb (500 g) total weight, peeled and chopped

This pairing of sweet potatoes and pungent parsnips and turnips is surprisingly delicious. The potato softens the bitterness of the other vegetables, making a delectable side dish for baked fish fillets or roast chicken.

In a saucepan, combine the parsnips, garlic, and broth. Cover and bring to a boil over high heat. Reduce the heat to low and simmer for 5 minutes. Carefully add the sweet potatoes and turnips, return to a simmer, and cook until all the vegetables are tender, 12–15 minutes.

Drain the vegetables in a colander placed over a large bowl to contain the broth. Return the vegetables to the pan. Carefully add ½ cup (4 fl oz/ 125 ml) of the hot cooking liquid to the vegetables. Using a potato masher or handheld mixer, mash the vegetables until light and fluffy. Add more of the broth, 1 tablespoon at a time, if necessary, for the desired consistency. Discard the remaining broth. Serve immediately.

NUTRIENT ANALYSIS FOR ONE SERVING

Calories from Fat 2%	**Calories from Carbs** 90%	**Total Fat** <1 g
Protein 3 g	**Carbohydrates** 34 g	**Saturated Fat** 0 g
Sodium 116 mg	**Fiber** 7 g	**Monounsaturated Fat** 0 g
Cholesterol 0 mg	**Sugars** 9 g	**Polyunsaturated Fat** 0 g

RED CABBAGE & APPLES WITH CARAWAY

SERVES 6

In this vibrant sweet-and-sour cabbage dish—a modern take on sauerkraut—the tartness of the vinegar plays off the sweetness of the apples. Serve with chicken or turkey sausages for a hearty dinner in fall or winter.

In a large, deep nonstick frying pan, heat the olive oil over medium heat. Add the onion and sauté until softened, about 5 minutes. Stir in the cabbage, apples, ½ cup broth, and caraway seeds. Raise the heat to medium-high, cover, and bring to a boil. Reduce the heat to low and simmer, covered, stirring occasionally, until the cabbage is tender, about 20 minutes. If all the liquid evaporates before the cabbage is done, stir in additional broth, ¼ cup (2 fl oz/60 ml) at a time. Stir in the vinegar and pepper and serve immediately.

1 teaspoon olive oil

1 small yellow onion, chopped

1 head red cabbage, about 2 lb (1 kg), trimmed, cored, and thinly sliced (about 8 cups/24 oz/750 g)

2 Granny Smith apples, peeled, cored, and chopped

½ cup (4 fl oz/125 ml) fat-free, no-salt-added vegetable or chicken broth, or as needed

¼ teaspoon caraway seeds

2 tablespoons red wine vinegar

¼ teaspoon freshly ground pepper

NUTRIENT ANALYSIS FOR ONE SERVING

Calories from Fat 11%	**Calories from Carbs** 79%	**Total Fat** 1 g
Protein 2 g	**Carbohydrates** 17 g	**Saturated Fat** 0 g
Sodium 61 mg	**Fiber** 3 g	**Monounsaturated Fat** 1 g
Cholesterol 0 mg	**Sugars** 10 g	**Polyunsaturated Fat** 0 g

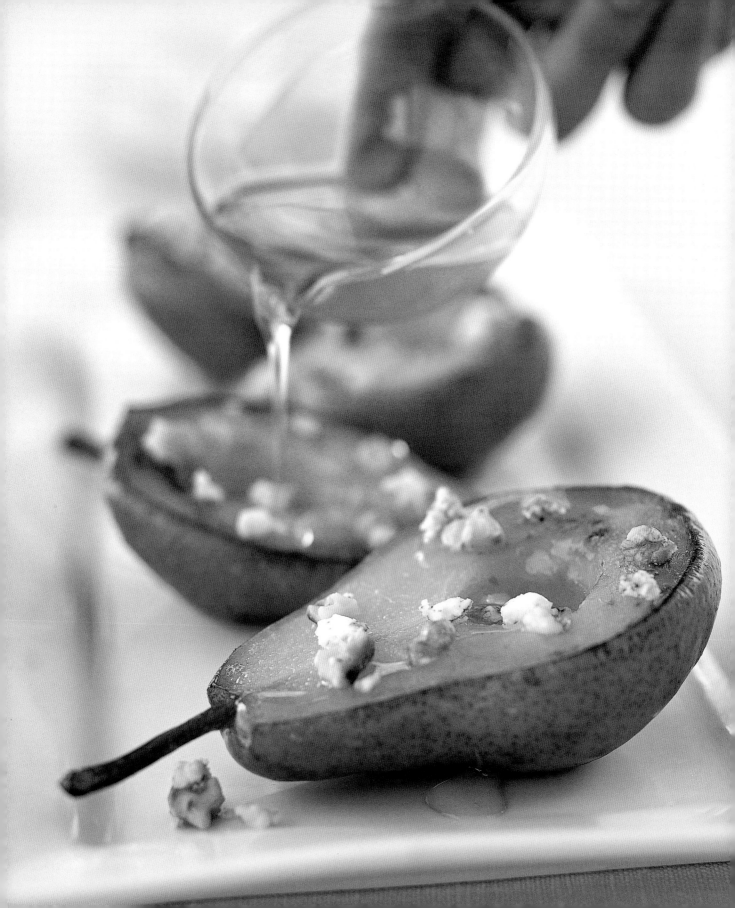

DESSERTS & SNACKS

52c WATERMELON POPS, 121

69c GRILLED PINEAPPLE WITH
ORANGE-CINNAMON GLAZE, 124

92c MELON SLICES WITH
RASPBERRY SAUCE, 129

98c ROASTED PEACHES WITH
GINGER SYRUP, 132

101c BANANA-BERRY PARFAITS, 118

112c BAKED PEARS WITH HONEY,
BLUE CHEESE & WALNUTS, 127

134c SPICED NECTARINE–BLUEBERRY
FRUIT SALAD, 133

139c CITRUS & RASPBERRIES
IN ORANGE SAUCE, 130

187c FRUIT & NUT TRAIL MIX, 122

188c BAKED STUFFED APPLES, 123

Baked Pears with Honey, Blue Cheese & Walnuts, 127

DIABETIC EXCHANGES

| 0 starch | 1 fruit | ½ milk |
| 0 vegetable | 0 protein | 0 fat |

BANANA-BERRY PARFAITS

SERVES 4   Kid-friendly recipe

1 cup (4 oz/125 g) strawberries, hulled and coarsely chopped

1 cup (8 oz/250 g) plain low-fat yogurt

1 banana, thinly sliced

1 cup (4 oz/125 g) blackberries

½ cup (2 oz/60 g) raspberries

The combination of fresh fruit and plain yogurt is a huge improvement in flavor over purchased fruit yogurts. This recipe uses strawberries, but try it with peaches or mangos. And with no added sugar, this dessert has diabetes-fighting benefits, too.

Place the strawberries in a bowl and mash with a fork or potato masher until crushed. Add the yogurt and stir to combine.

To assemble each parfait, spoon about 3 tablespoons of the yogurt mixture into a wineglass. Top the yogurt with one-fourth of the banana slices. Then spoon another 3 tablespoons of the yogurt mixture over the banana. Top with ¼ cup (1 oz/30 g) of the blackberries and one-fourth of the raspberries. Repeat to make 3 more parfaits.

Serve the parfaits immediately, or cover with plastic wrap and refrigerate for up to 2 hours. Let stand for 20 minutes at room temperature before serving.

NUTRIENT ANALYSIS FOR ONE SERVING

Calories from Fat 11%	**Calories from Carbs** 73%	**Total Fat** 1 g
Protein 4 g	**Carbohydrates** 20 g	**Saturated Fat** 1 g
Sodium 44 mg	**Fiber** 3 g	**Monounsaturated Fat** 0 g
Cholesterol 4 mg	**Sugars** 12 g	**Polyunsaturated Fat** 0 g

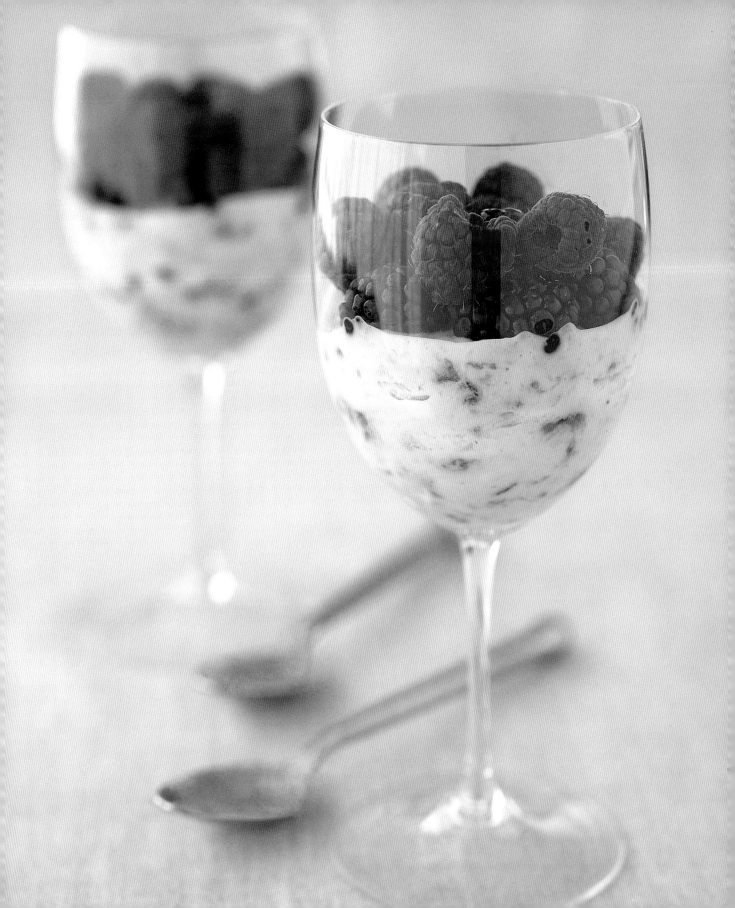

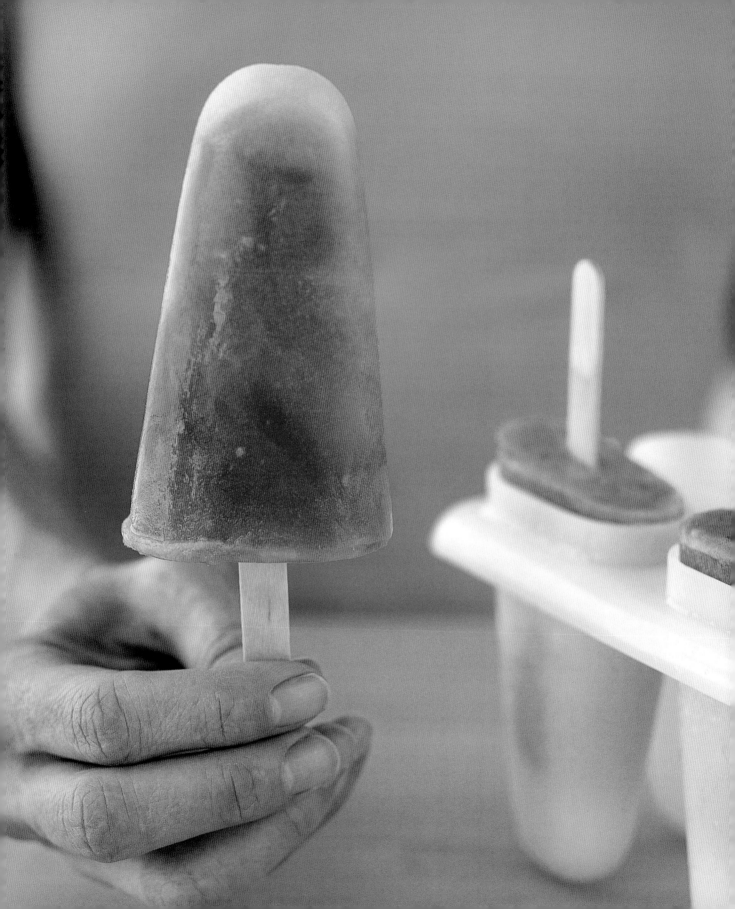

WATERMELON POPS

DIABETIC EXCHANGES
| 0 starch | 1 fruit | 0 milk |
| 0 vegetable | 0 protein | 0 fat |

SERVES 6   Kid-friendly recipe

Please the children with a hot-pink pop that's practically free of calories but full of fun. You can also purée the frozen cubes in a food processor to make a stunning sorbet to serve at the end of an elegant dinner.

In a food processor, combine the watermelon cubes and the lime juice and process until smooth. Pour the watermelon mixture into popsicle molds or into small paper cups and freeze until slushy, about 2 hours. Insert popsicle sticks and freeze until firm, at least 6 hours longer.

Alternatively, freeze the watermelon-lime mixture in ice cube trays. Let the cubes soften slightly at room temperature and serve in deep-sided bowls with spoons. The pops or cubes will keep for up to 1 week in the freezer.

4 cups (1½ lb/750 g) 1-inch (2.5-cm) cubes seedless watermelon

1 tablespoon fresh lime juice

NUTRIENT ANALYSIS FOR ONE SERVING

Calories from Fat 4%	Calories from Carbs 89%	Total Fat <1 g
Protein 1 g	Carbohydrates 13 g	Saturated Fat 0 g
Sodium 2 mg	Fiber 1 g	Monounsaturated Fat 0 g
Cholesterol 0 mg	Sugars 11 g	Polyunsaturated Fat 0 g

FRUIT & NUT TRAIL MIX

DIABETIC EXCHANGES

½ starch	2 fruit	0 milk
0 vegetable	½ protein	½ fat

SERVES 6

Kid-friendly recipe

1 cup (2 oz/60 g) spoon-size shredded wheat and/or bran cereal

⅛ teaspoon ground cinnamon

1 cup (3 oz/90 g) dried apple slices, halved

½ cup (1½ oz/45 g) dried peaches, halved

½ cup (3 oz/90 g) raisins

¼ cup unsalted dry roasted peanuts

Tuck this mix into kids' lunch boxes for a super-healthy, fiber-loaded school snack. Make a double batch to keep on hand when little ones—or adults—need a mid-afternoon treat that's filling, nourishing, and fun to eat.

Preheat the oven to 350°F (180°C).

In a bowl, combine the cereal and cinnamon and toss to coat. Arrange the cereal in a single layer on a rimmed baking sheet. Bake until lightly toasted and crisp, 5–7 minutes. Transfer the pan to a wire rack and let the mix cool to room temperature.

In a bowl, combine the toasted cereal, apples, peaches, raisins, and peanuts and toss to distribute the ingredients evenly. Store tightly covered at room temperature for up to 1 week.

NUTRIENT ANALYSIS FOR ONE SERVING

Calories from Fat 15%	Calories from Carbs 78%	Total Fat 3 g
Protein 4 g	Carbohydrates 40 g	Saturated Fat 0 g
Sodium 157 mg	Fiber 5 g	Monounsaturated Fat 2 g
Cholesterol 0 mg	Sugars 25 g	Polyunsaturated Fat 1 g

BAKED STUFFED APPLES

SERVES 4

Cutting away a ribbon of peel around the center of apples before baking ensures that they keep their shape. If you can't find Rome apples, use Gala, Braeburn, or Gravenstein. Any mixture of dried fruits and nuts will work in this recipe.

Preheat the oven to 350°F (180°C).

In a small bowl, combine the raisins, apricots, pecans, cinnamon, and nutmeg. Stir to mix well. Set aside.

Working from the stem end, cut the core from each apple, stopping ½ inch (12 mm) from the bottom. Peel away a ½-inch (12-mm) strip of skin around the circumference of each apple at the center. Divide the dried fruit mixture evenly among the apples, pressing the mixture gently into each cavity.

Arrange the apples upright in a small baking dish just large enough to hold them. Pour the apple cider into the dish. Cover the dish snugly with aluminum foil. Bake until the apples are tender when pierced with a knife, 25–30 minutes.

To serve, transfer one apple to each of 4 bowls and drizzle each apple with the pan juices. Serve warm or at room temperature.

⅓ cup (2 oz/60 g) golden raisins (sultanas)

4 dried apricots, diced

2 tablespoons chopped pecans

¼ teaspoon ground cinnamon

⅛ teaspoon freshly ground nutmeg

4 Rome apples, about 1½ lb (750 g) total weight

½ cup (4 fl oz/125 ml) apple cider

NUTRIENT ANALYSIS FOR ONE SERVING

Calories from Fat 12%	**Calories from Carbs** 86%	**Total Fat** 3 g
Protein 1 g	**Carbohydrates** 44 g	**Saturated Fat** 0 g
Sodium 10 mg	**Fiber** 7 g	**Monounsaturated Fat** 2 g
Cholesterol 0 mg	**Sugars** 32 g	**Polyunsaturated Fat** 1 g

GRILLED PINEAPPLE WITH ORANGE-CINNAMON GLAZE

SERVES 4   Kid-friendly recipe

½ cup (4 fl oz/125 ml) fresh orange juice

¼ teaspoon ground cinnamon

1 firm but ripe pineapple, about 3 lb (1.5 kg)

If you don't feel like peeling a pineapple, look for fresh pineapple already peeled and cored. You'll find it in plastic containers in the supermarket produce section. You'll need about 32 oz (1 kg) of prepared pineapple.

Prepare a fire in a charcoal grill or preheat a gas grill or oven broiler. Lightly coat the grill rack or broiler pan with olive oil cooking spray. Position the grill rack or broiler pan 4–6 inches (10–15 cm) from the heat source.

In a bowl, whisk together the orange juice and cinnamon. Set aside.

Cut off the crown of leaves and the base of the pineapple. Stand the pineapple upright and, using a large, sharp knife, pare off the skin, cutting downward just below the surface in long vertical strips and leaving the small brown "eyes" on the fruit. Lay the pineapple on its side. Aligning the knife blade with the diagonal rows of eyes, cut a shallow furrow, following a spiral pattern around the pineapple, to remove all the eyes. Cut the pineapple into eight ½-inch (12-mm) slices. Place each slice on a cutting board and use an apple corer to cut away the core of each slice.

Lightly brush the pineapple with the orange juice mixture. Grill or broil, turning once and basting once or twice with the glaze, until tender and golden, about 3 minutes on each side. Transfer to a platter or individual plates. Serve hot or warm.

NUTRIENT ANALYSIS FOR ONE SERVING

Calories from Fat 2%	**Calories from Carbs** 93%	**Total Fat** <1 g
Protein 1 g	**Carbohydrates** 18 g	**Saturated Fat** 0 g
Sodium 1 mg	**Fiber** 2 g	**Monounsaturated Fat** 0 g
Cholesterol 0 mg	**Sugars** 13 g	**Polyunsaturated Fat** 0 g

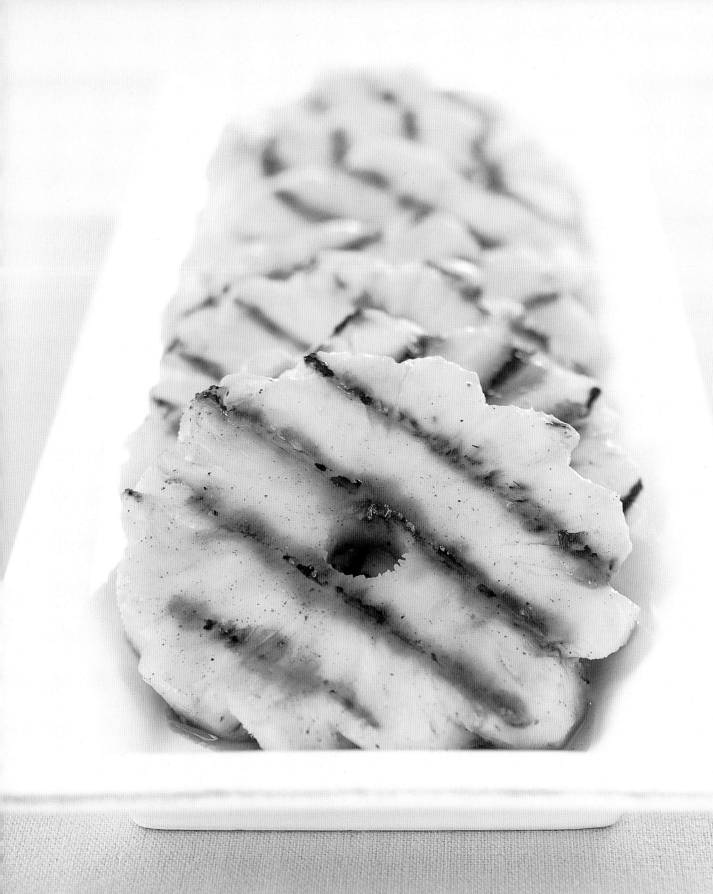

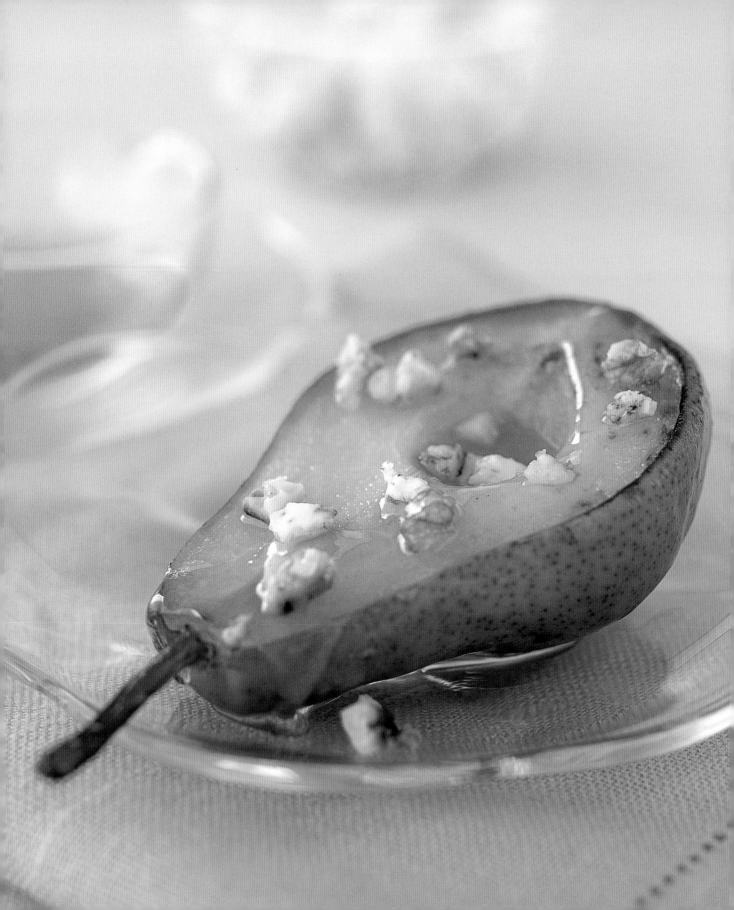

BAKED PEARS WITH HONEY, BLUE CHEESE & WALNUTS

SERVES 4

The success of this simple but sophisticated dessert depends on using pears that aren't too ripe—choose fruit that is still firm to the touch. For a more casual meal, serve the pears alone or topped with plain yogurt and drizzled with honey.

Preheat the oven to 450°F (230°C).

Coat a shallow roasting pan or rimmed baking sheet with the olive oil. Cut the pears in half and use a melon baller to remove the cores. Place the pears, cut side down, in the prepared pan. Bake until the pears are tender and the cut sides are lightly browned, about 20 minutes.

While the pears are baking, put the walnuts in a small, dry, nonstick frying pan over medium-low heat. Cook, stirring constantly, until lightly toasted, about 2 minutes. Transfer to a plate and set aside.

To serve, place each pear half, cut side up, on an individual plate. Sprinkle each with the toasted walnuts and blue cheese, and drizzle with the honey. Serve warm or at room temperature.

1 teaspoon olive oil

2 firm but ripe Bartlett pears

1 tablespoon chopped walnuts

1 tablespoon crumbled blue cheese

2 tablespoons honey

NUTRIENT ANALYSIS FOR ONE SERVING

Calories from Fat 26%	**Calories from Carbs** 70%	**Total Fat** 4 g
Protein 1 g	**Carbohydrates** 22 g	**Saturated Fat** 1 g
Sodium 30 mg	**Fiber** 2 g	**Monounsaturated Fat** 1 g
Cholesterol 2 mg	**Sugars** 17 g	**Polyunsaturated Fat** 1 g

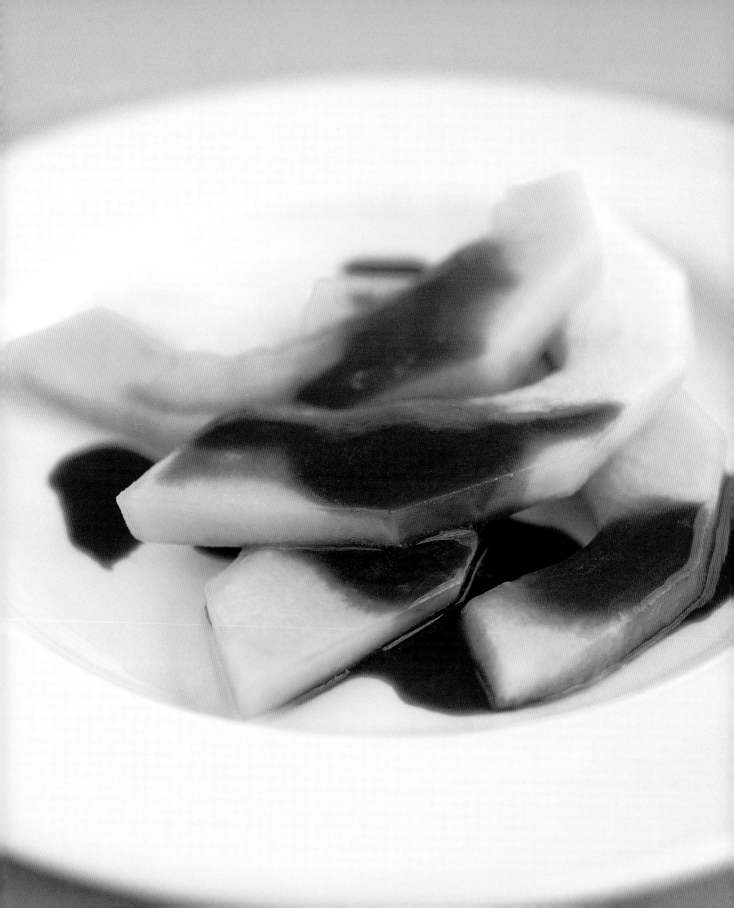

MELON SLICES WITH RASPBERRY SAUCE

CALORIES

92

DIABETIC EXCHANGES

| 0 starch | 1½ fruit | 0 milk |
| 0 vegetable | 0 protein | 0 fat |

SERVES 4

To make the sauce, make sure the frozen raspberries are completely thawed so they'll be easier to purée. The raspberry sauce is delicious on any kind of fresh fruit; try it on bananas or pineapple, or drizzle it over plain yogurt.

Place the raspberries in a food processor or blender and purée until smooth. Pass the purée through a fine-mesh sieve placed over a bowl, pressing firmly on the solids with a rubber spatula or the back of a wooden spoon to extract all the juice. Scrape the inside of the sieve periodically to dislodge any seeds that may be plugging the holes. Keep pushing the pulp firmly through the sieve until all that is left is a small number of seeds. Cover the purée and refrigerate until ready to use.

Using a spoon, remove and discard the seeds from the melon halves. Using a sharp knife, cut away the peel. Cut the flesh into thin slices.

To serve, divide the melon slices among individual plates and drizzle with the raspberry sauce.

One 10-oz (315-g) package frozen raspberries, thawed

½ small cantaloupe, about 2 lb (1 kg)

½ small honeydew melon, about 2½ lb (1.25 kg)

NUTRIENT ANALYSIS FOR ONE SERVING

Calories from Fat 3%	Calories from Carbs 89%	Total Fat <1 g
Protein 2 g	Carbohydrates 22 g	Saturated Fat 0 g
Sodium 31 mg	Fiber 1 g	Monounsaturated Fat 0 g
Cholesterol 0 mg	Sugars 13 g	Polyunsaturated Fat 0 g

CITRUS & RASPBERRIES IN ORANGE SAUCE

SERVES 4

- 1 cup (8 fl oz/ 250 ml) fresh orange juice
- ⅛ teaspoon vanilla extract (essence)
- 2 large navel oranges
- 2 pink grapefruits
- 1 cup (4 oz/125 g) raspberries
- 4 fresh mint sprigs (optional)

If you have time, drizzle the citrus slices with the sauce and let them stand for an hour at room temperature before serving so the fruit will absorb the vanilla and orange flavors. Use Ruby grapefruits to make this vitamin C–packed treat even sweeter.

In a saucepan over medium heat, bring the orange juice to a boil. Reduce the heat to low and simmer, uncovered, until reduced to ⅓ cup (3 fl oz/ 80 ml), about 8 minutes. Set aside and let cool to room temperature. Stir in the vanilla.

While the orange juice is simmering, segment the citrus fruits: Working with one orange or grapefruit at a time, cut a thin slice off the top and the bottom, exposing the flesh. Stand the fruit upright and, using a sharp knife, cut off the peel in thick strips, following the contour of the fruit and removing all the white pith and membrane. Cut the fruit crosswise into slices ½ inch (12 mm) thick. Repeat with the remaining citrus fruit.

To serve, divide the citrus slices among individual plates. Top with the raspberries. Drizzle each serving with about 1 tablespoon of the orange sauce. Garnish with the mint, if desired.

NUTRIENT ANALYSIS FOR ONE SERVING

Calories from Fat 2%	**Calories from Carbs** 92%	**Total Fat** 0 g
Protein 2 g	**Carbohydrates** 37 g	**Saturated Fat** 0 g
Sodium 1 mg	**Fiber** 12 g	**Monounsaturated Fat** 0 g
Cholesterol 0 mg	**Sugars** 24 g	**Polyunsaturated Fat** 0 g

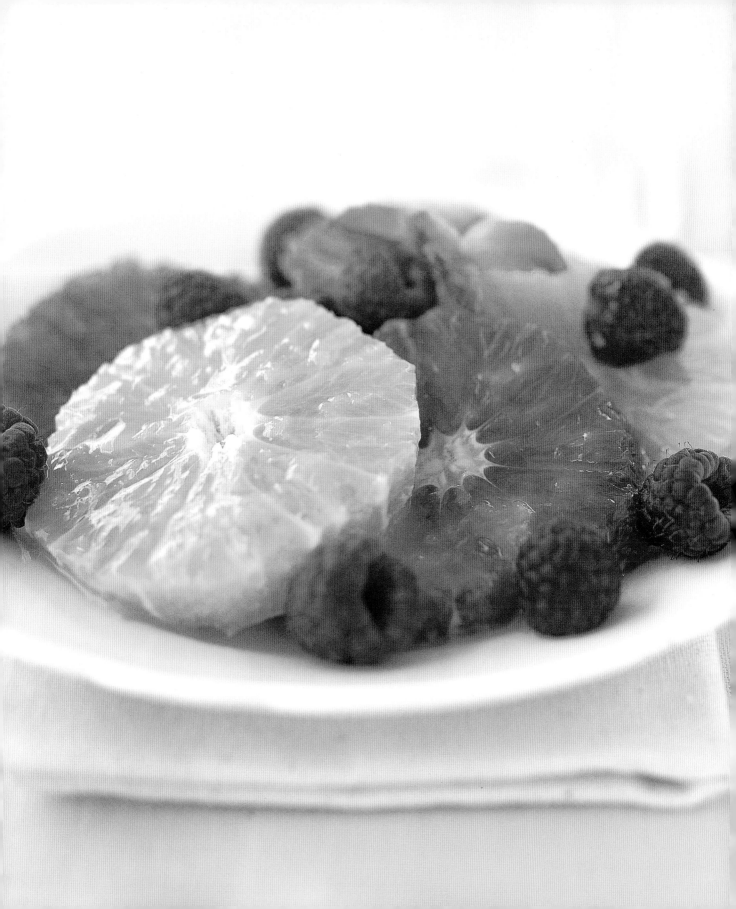

ROASTED PEACHES WITH GINGER SYRUP

SERVES 4

1 teaspoon olive oil

4 peaches, about 1½ lb (750 g) total weight, peel intact, cut in half and pitted

1½ cups (12 fl oz/375 ml) peach nectar

1 tablespoon peeled and minced fresh ginger

Roasting caramelizes peaches and concentrates their flavor. Choose freestone peach varieties, because their fruit separates more easily from the pit. If peaches are unavailable, nectarines work just as well.

Preheat the oven to 450°F (230°C).

Coat a shallow roasting pan or rimmed baking sheet with the olive oil. Place the peaches, cut side down, in the pan. Bake until the peaches are tender and the cut sides are lightly browned, about 20 minutes.

While the peaches are baking, combine the peach nectar and ginger in a saucepan and bring to a boil over medium heat. Reduce the heat to low and simmer, uncovered, until reduced to ½ cup (4 fl oz/125 ml), 8–10 minutes. Pour the mixture through a fine-mesh sieve placed over a bowl. Discard the solids remaining in the sieve. Set the syrup aside.

To serve, place 2 peach halves in each of 4 bowls and drizzle each serving with about 2 tablespoons of the syrup. Serve warm or at room temperature.

NUTRIENT ANALYSIS FOR ONE SERVING

Calories from Fat 10%	**Calories from Carbs** 85%	**Total Fat** 1 g
Protein 1 g	**Carbohydrates** 23 g	**Saturated Fat** 0 g
Sodium 6 mg	**Fiber** 3 g	**Monounsaturated Fat** 1 g
Cholesterol 0 mg	**Sugars** 20 g	**Polyunsaturated Fat** 0 g

SPICED NECTARINE-BLUEBERRY FRUIT SALAD

DIABETIC EXCHANGES

0 starch	2 fruit	0 milk
0 vegetable	0 protein	0 fat

SERVES 4

In the dressing for this dessert salad, whole spices infuse their comforting aroma and lively flavor into the apple juice as it simmers down to a delicious syrup. Drizzle it over pancakes or fresh fruit salad, or add a splash to a glass of iced tea.

In a saucepan, combine the apple juice, cloves, star anise, and cinnamon stick and bring to a boil over medium heat. Reduce the heat to low and simmer, uncovered, until the juice is reduced to ½ cup (4 fl oz/125 ml), about 15 minutes. Pour the mixture through a fine-mesh sieve placed over a bowl. Discard the spices. Set aside to cool.

To serve, arrange one of the sliced nectarines and ¼ cup (1 oz/30 g) of the blueberries in each of 4 bowls. Drizzle each serving with about 2 tablespoons of the spiced apple juice.

1½ cups (12 fl oz/375 ml) unsweetened apple juice

¼ teaspoon whole cloves

2 whole star anise

One 3-inch (7.5-cm) cinnamon stick

4 nectarines, peel intact, pitted and sliced

1 cup (4 oz/125 g) blueberries

NUTRIENT ANALYSIS FOR ONE SERVING

Calories from Fat 5%	**Calories from Carbs** 92%	**Total Fat** 1 g
Protein 1 g	**Carbohydrates** 32 g	**Saturated Fat** 0 g
Sodium 3 mg	**Fiber** 3 g	**Monounsaturated Fat** 0 g
Cholesterol 0 mg	**Sugars** 26 g	**Polyunsaturated Fat** 0 g

INGREDIENTS & TECHNIQUES

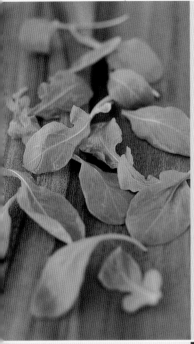

ARUGULA

Also known as rocket, this leafy salad green has a tangy, peppery taste. Its markedly notched leaves resemble elongated oak leaves, and measure about 3 inches (7.5 cm) in length. Buy bunches with bright green leaves and no signs of wilting. Remove any thick stem ends before using. Bunches should be stored in a tightly sealed plastic bag in the refrigerator and used within a day or two.

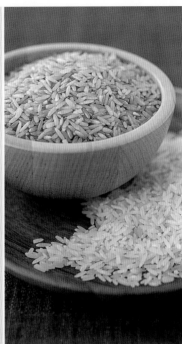

BROWN RICE

Brown rice has not been processed by milling or polishing. Its brown hull is still intact, thus retaining the grain's fiber, B vitamins, minerals, and oils. Brown rice takes longer to cook than white rice and it has a chewier texture and more robust taste. Short-, medium-, and long-grain varieties are available. Store in an airtight container and use within 6 months, or for up to 1 year if refrigerated.

BARLEY

This grain—which has been cultivated for almost 8,000 years—is most popularly used in soups today. However, its nutty flavor and chewy texture lend themselves to many delicious preparations. Try barley cooked risotto-style, added to stews, and cold in salads. The most commonly used variety is pearl barley, which is hulled and polished to a pearl-like sheen.

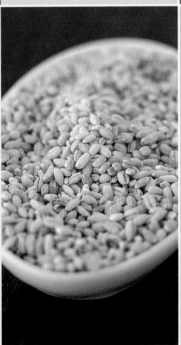

BULGUR WHEAT

A staple in the Middle East, bulgur comes from whole wheat kernels that have been partially steamed, dried, and then cracked. It is widely available in a range of granulations, from a coarse grain for pilaf to a fine grinding for tabbouleh. Commonly used in salads, soups, and fillings, bulgur requires only brief soaking in water or a few minutes of cooking to bring out its nutty flavor.

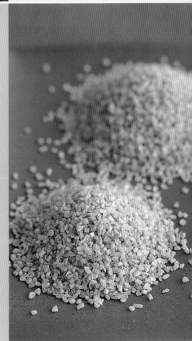

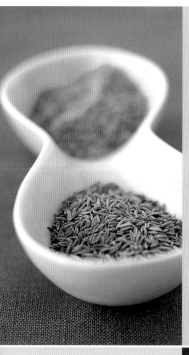

CUMIN

The seeds of a member of the parsley family, cumin has a sharp, strong flavor perfect for use in assertive dishes. Cumin is available both ground and whole. For superior flavor, buy whole light-brown seeds and toast them before grinding for use as needed. All spices, including cumin, should be stored in tightly covered containers in a cool, dark place. They will keep for up to 1 year.

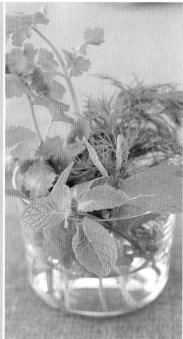

HERBS

Choose fresh herbs that look bright and healthy, and are fragrant. Avoid any that have wilted or discolored leaves. Fresh herbs should be refrigerated in sealed plastic bags. Buy dried herbs in small amounts and store them in tightly covered glass jars. Since dried herbs have more concentrated flavors, use one-fourth the amount of the fresh version called for.

GINGER

Gnarled and knobby in appearance, fresh ginger has a thin brown skin that is easy to remove with a paring knife or vegetable peeler. It has a refreshing and slightly sweet flavor that is also quite spicy. Select heavy pieces that are firm and smooth with slightly shiny skin. Store it unpeeled in a sealed plastic bag in the refrigerator for up to 3 weeks or in the freezer for up to 1 year.

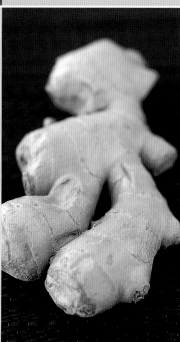

KALE & CHARD

Kale has firm, dark green, lightly crinkled leaves on long stems. This member of the cabbage family is rich in vitamins A and B and the minerals calcium and iron. It retains its texture well when cooked. Chard, also known as Swiss chard, has large, crinkled leaves on white stems. Red chard has a more earthy flavor than the white kind, which tends to taste somewhat sweet.

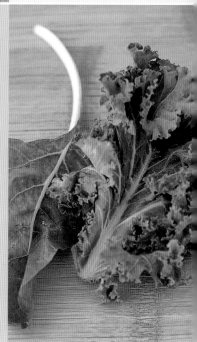

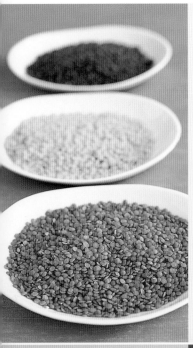

LENTILS

A staple in the Middle East for 8,000 years, lentils are available in dozens of types grown around the world. Varieties include the common brown lentil found in most supermarkets, dark green Le Puy lentils from France, yellow lentils from India, and the small red lentils of Egypt. Although always dried, they do not require presoaking and cook to tenderness in only 20 to 30 minutes.

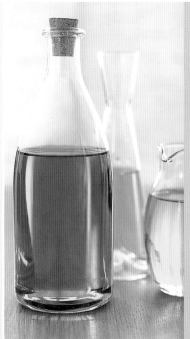

OLIVE OIL

Essential to Mediterranean cuisine, olive oils can be bright green and peppery or mellow gold and slightly sweet. Extra-virgin olive oil, the highest quality grade, retains the most color and flavor, but it is best reserved for sauces and quick sautés, as it loses character at even moderate temperatures. Regular olive oil, lighter in flavor and color, holds up well to high-heat cooking such as frying.

NUTMEG

Native to Indonesia, nutmeg has a warm, sweet-spicy flavor that marries well with spinach, fish, meat fillings, milk-based dishes, and many desserts. Because its aromatic oils dissipate quickly once the seed is ground, try to use whole nutmeg whenever possible. Although special nutmeg graters ensure the finest shavings, any type of fine-holed grater will work well for this purpose.

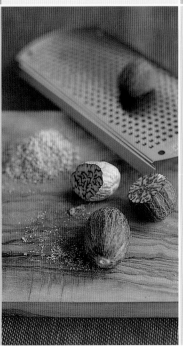

PARMIGIANO-REGGIANO

This trademarked aged cow's-milk cheese is named for the Italian provinces of Parma and Reggio Emilia and is renowned for its complex and appealing flavor. As it tastes quite salty, a small amount can add great depth of taste to a dish, especially when the cheese is top-quality, purchased in block form, and grated by hand just before serving.

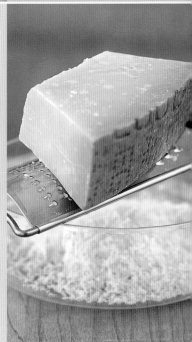

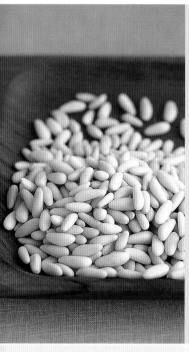

PINE NUTS

Also known as pignoli or piñon nuts, these pale, slender nuts are laboriously harvested from the cones of pine trees indigenous to the forests of southern Europe and the southern United States. Ground or whole, they lend richness to a wide variety of savory and sweet dishes, from classic Italian pesto and Mexican sweets to simple salads and pastas. They're especially good toasted.

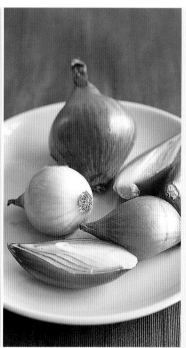

SHALLOTS

Diminutive members of the onion family, shallots grow in small clusters much like garlic. Their papery reddish brown skin covers white flesh tinged with pink or purple. Although layered like onions, with a similar pungent aroma, they are valued for their more delicate flavor, which is particularly good in sauces and vinaigrettes. Store shallots in a cool, dark place with good air circulation.

SESAME OIL

Made from toasted sesame seeds, dark sesame oil has a rich amber color and an intense, nutty flavor. Clear, refined sesame oils are better for high-heat cooking, but dark oils offer more flavor, even in tiny amounts. Look for them in Asian markets or the ethnic or international aisle of supermarkets. More perishable than other oils, dark sesame oil is best stored in the refrigerator.

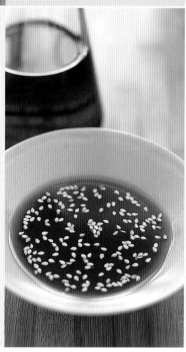

SOYBEANS, FRESH

Also known as edamame, soybeans picked still in their pods retain a bright green color and a fresh, nutty flavor. Left whole, they can be boiled or steamed for a snack. Shelled, they're enjoyed like English peas in vegetable dishes, soups, or purées. Look for soybeans during summer in produce markets or year-round in the freezers of natural-food stores, Asian markets, and many large supermarkets.

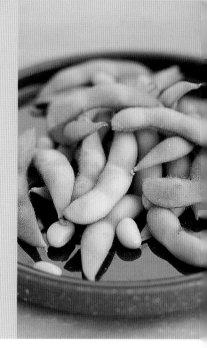

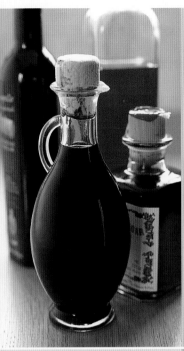

SPECIALTY VINEGARS

From the French for "sour wine," vinegar forms when bacteria turn a fermented liquid into a weak solution of acetic acid. Red wine, white wine, balsamic, and sherry vinegars are among the best for cooking, as they display traits of the wines from which they are made, along with a sourness that makes them valuable in balancing flavors. Look for top-quality, unfiltered aged vinegars.

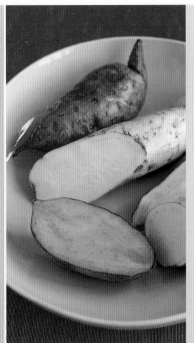

SWEET POTATOES

Although often confused with yams, sweet potatoes have a sweeter flavor and less starchy flesh. They are excellent baked whole, roasted or braised with a honey or maple syrup glaze, or mashed with a touch of cinnamon or nutmeg. Shop for sweet potatoes free of dark blemishes. Store in a cool, dark, well-ventilated place but avoid refrigerating them, as cold temperatures will alter their flavor.

SUN-DRIED TOMATOES

Dehydrated plum tomatoes are available either dried (labeled "dry packed") or packed in oil. The dry-packed variety must be reconstituted for about 5 minutes in hot water before using. They contain almost no fat (compared with oil-packed tomatoes) and are naturally low in calories and sodium. All tomatoes are rich in the antioxidant vitamins A and C, as well as lycopene.

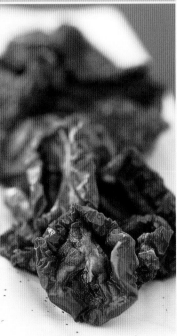

TOASTING NUTS

Cooking nuts until they are golden deepens their flavor and improves their texture. You can toast nuts by baking them on a cookie sheet in a 325°F (165°C) oven or by stirring them in a small, dry, nonstick frying pan over medium-high heat. Cook them just until they're fragrant and golden in color, about 5–10 minutes. Take care not to overcook them, as they will become bitter when scorched.

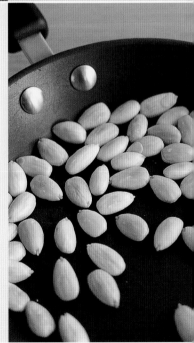

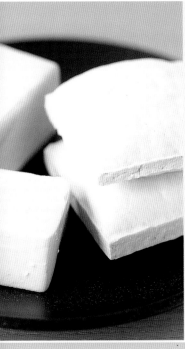

TOFU

Soy milk, made from cooked soybeans, forms tofu when curdled and pressed into blocks. Although bland, plain tofu readily absorbs flavors from marinades and sauces. The smooth texture of silken tofu is ideal for soups and for puréeing. Firm tofu, denser and coarser in texture, holds together well for stir-frying and grilling. To store tofu, submerge it in cold water and refrigerate.

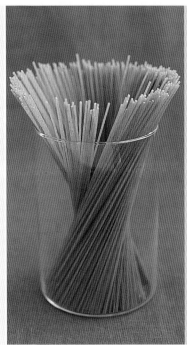

WHOLE-WHEAT NOODLES

Whole-wheat noodles, available in health food shops and well-stocked grocery stores, add a delicious and fiber-packed punch to your favorite pasta dishes. They are made from whole, unrefined grains, which still have their outer layers of bran and germ intact. As a result, whole-wheat noodles are rich in vitamin E and are healthy for the heart.

VINAIGRETTE

Making a vinaigrette involves little more than whisking together a small amount of oil, vinegar, salt, pepper, and perhaps an aromatic ingredient such as garlic, shallots, a dab of prepared mustard, or some minced fresh herbs. In addition to dressing salads, a vinaigrette can be used as a marinade before roasting, a basting liquid at the grill, or a sauce for steamed vegetables.

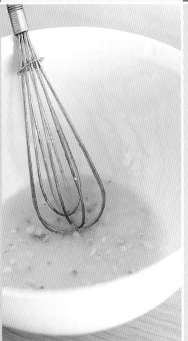

ZEST

The thin outer peel of citrus fruits, known as the zest, is rich in aromatic oils. You can use any type of fine-holed grater to shred the zest into delicate shavings for marinades or rubs. Use a zester to create thin, elegant strips for garnish. Take care not to cut or grate into the white, pulpy pith that lies just beneath the outer peel, as it has a spongy texture and an unpleasantly bitter flavor.

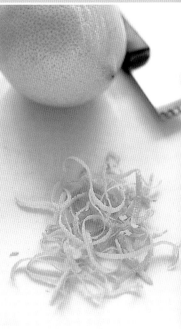

INDEX

WELDON OWEN INC.

Chief Executive Officer: John Owen

President and Chief Operating Officer: Terry Newell

Chief Financial Officer: Christine E. Munson

Vice President International Sales: Stuart Laurence

Creative Director: Gaye Allen

Associate Publisher: Val Cipollone

Editor: Emily Miller

Contributing Editor: Sheridan Warrick

Designer: Leon Yu

Editorial Assistant: Juli Vendzules

Copy Editor: Carrie Bradley

Proofreaders: Arin Hailey and Sharron Wood

Indexer: Ken DellaPenta

Production Director: Chris Hemesath

Color Manager: Teri Bell

Production and Reprint Coordinator: Todd Rechner

The Type 2 Diabetes Cookbook

Conceived and produced by Weldon Owen Inc.

814 Montgomery Street, San Francisco, CA 94133

Telephone: 415-291-0100 Fax: 415-291-8841

First printed in 2005

10 9 8 7 6 5 4 3 2 1

ISBN: 1-74089-539-8

Printed by Midas Printing Limited, China

Acknowledgments

Thanks to Nicky Collings, Joan Olsen, and Colin Wheatland for
design assistance; Kim Konecny and Erin Quon for food styling;
Leigh Noë for prop styling; Selena Aument and Guarina Lopez for
studio assistance; and models Nancy, Eric E., and Robert J. Wong.

Photographs by Jim Franco: page 12, page 13 (three at top right
corner), page 14 (three at top left corner), page 16 (three at top left
corner), page 17 (top), page 19, page 134 (bottom right), page 136
(three at left), page 137.